Working in Care Settings

Val Michie

Published in 2004 by:
Nelson Thornes Ltd
Delta Place
27 Bath Road
CHELTENHAM
GL53 7TH
United Kingdom

04 05 06 07 08 / 10 9 8 7 6 5 4 3 2

A catalogue record for this book is available from the British Library

ISBN 0-7487-7483-1

Illustrations by Clinton Banbury and Angela Lumley
Page make-up by Northern Phototypesetting Co Ltd, Bolton

Printed in Great Britain by Ashford Colour Press

Acknowledgements

I have been inspired by numerous people and situations to write this book, but in particular I would like to acknowledge:

Bubbles Higgins and Mary Michie, for their experiences of being cared for. All my students, past and present, for their experiences as care workers. Sue Shotton, Chris Howey and Sue Thompson for their expert technical advice and guidance.

Julia Pilling, for her invaluable feedback and suggestions and Tony Michie, for his enduring support and countless cups of coffee!

I would also like to thank Helen Broadfield and Helen Kerindi at Nelson Thornes for all their hard work.

Contents

Introduction

Why read this book?

Everybody who starts to work with older people to help meet their care needs must receive training to a certain standard. Within their first 6 weeks of employment they must receive Induction Standards training. Within their first 6 months of employment they must receive Foundation Standards training. The point of Induction and Foundation Standards training is to help care workers develop the knowledge and understanding that support good working practices.

The reading material in this book covers the knowledge and understanding that you need to complete your induction and foundation training:

- Chapters 1–5 cover what you need to know and understand for your Induction Standards training
- Chapters 6–10 build on the first five chapters and cover what you need to know and understand for your Foundation Standards training.

The reading material also provides much of the underpinning knowledge and understanding needed for a number of Care NVQ units. These are highlighted at the beginning of each chapter. In addition, completing the activities gives you the chance to develop your discussion, reading and writing skills and to build your portfolio for the key skill qualification Communication at level 1.

How to achieve the Induction and Foundation Standards

This book has been written in a style and at a level that will appeal to you if you have not had recent experience of learning or if you are not confident in your ability to learn.

The activities throughout the book are linked to the TOPSS England Induction and Foundation Standards and give you the opportunity to think about, check and demonstrate your knowledge and understanding.

Case studies focus what you are learning into a practical situation that you may experience at work. They help you to imagine what you would do if you were involved in the issue being presented.

What do you think? encourages you to reflect on what you've just read, or think about the way you work.

Develop good work practice invites you to concentrate on your workplace, looking at procedures and the way you work with your service users and colleagues. Can these be improved?

Check your understanding is a way for you to make sure you have understood the topics you've just read.

Completing the activities will provide the evidence you need to achieve the Standards.

The book has been written primarily to support care workers who work with elderly people. However, it also provides much of the knowledge and understanding needed if you work with adults and young people who have disabilities and learning difficulties.

I hope you enjoy this book and that it helps you find achievement, fulfilment and success in your job. I also hope that it whets your appetite for further learning and self-development.

MAPPING GRID

Mapping of chapters and activities to TOPSS Induction and Foundation standards, Care NVQ level 2 units and and key skill Communication at level 1

Chapter Links to Care NVQ level 2 Units	Activity	Links to Induction/ Foundation standards	Links to key skill Communication level 1
1. Understanding the principles of care			
O1, CL1, CL2, CL5, CU5, Z1	1	Induction standard 1.1.1	C1.2
	2	Induction standard 1.1.2	C1.1 (1:1); C1.2
	3	Induction standard 1.2.1	C1.2
	4	Induction standard 1.2.2	C1.2
	5	Induction standard 1.2.3	C1.2
	6	Induction standard 1.3.1	C1.1 (1:1); C1.2
	7	Induction standard 1.4.1	C1.1 (1:1); C1.2
	8	Induction standard 1.4.2	C1.1 (1:1); C1.2
	9	Induction standard 1.4.3	C1.1 (1:1); C1.2
2. Understanding your workplace	10	Induction standard 2.1.1	C1.2
and your role as a worker	11	Induction standard 2.1.2	C1.1 (1:1); C1.2
O1, CU1, CU3, CU5, CU10, W2,	12	Induction standard 2.2.1	C1.1 (1:1); C1.2
W8, Z1, Z7	13	Induction standard 2.3.1	C1.2
	14	Induction standard 2.3.2	C1.1 (1:1); C1.2
	15	Induction standard 2.3.3	C1.2
	16	Induction standard 2.3.4	C1.2
	17	Induction standard 2.3.5	C1.1 (1:1); C1.2
3. Understanding the experiences	18	Induction standard 3.1.1	C1.2
and particular needs of service	19	Induction standard 3.1.2	C1.1 (1:1); C1.2
user groups	20	Induction standard 3.2.1	C1.1 (1:1); C1.2
O1, CL1, CL2, CL5,	21	Induction standard 3.2.2	C1.2
NC12, Z6, Z8, Z9, Z11, Z19	22	Induction standard 3.2.3	C1.1 (1:1); C1.2
	23	Induction standard 3.2.4	C1.1 (1:1); C1.2
	24	Induction standard 3.2.5	C1.1 (1:1); C1.2

1 Understanding the principles of care

The principles of care set the standards for how you should work with your colleagues, managers, people from other organisations and especially with service users and their families and friends. This chapter aims to develop your knowledge and understanding of the principles of care so that you can develop and use good day-to-day working practices.

Successful completion of the activities in this chapter will enable you to demonstrate your understanding of the Induction Standard *Understand the principles of care*. It will also give you an opportunity to develop evidence for key skills unit Communication at level 1.

What is covered in this chapter?

This chapter contributes to the knowledge and understanding you need for the following NVQ Care units:

- O1 : Foster people's equality, diversity and rights
- CL1 : Promote effective communication and relationships
- CL2 : Promote communication with individuals where there are communication differences
- CL5 : Promote communication with those who do not use a recognised language format
- CU5: Receive, transmit, store and retrieve information
- Z1 : Contribute to the protection of individuals from abuse

1.1 THE CARE VALUES

The care values are the beliefs that underpin care work. Using the care values in your work is good practice because it shows those you work with that you value them. There are a number of ways that you can show you value people in your work.

Showing respect

Showing someone respect shows that you value them for who they are. It also means that you consider them in what you do with and for them. Respect runs through all the care values.

Recognising individuality

Each of us has a unique set of genes and life experiences that have made us the way we are and that set us apart from everybody else. Although we have much in common with each other, even the closest friends and family members have different personalities, likes and dislikes, ways of doing things, beliefs and opinions.

Recognising and respecting people's individual differences in the way you work with them demonstrates that you value them. By treating people as individuals you will help them feel good about themselves, special and reassured that you understand them.

Respecting rights

Except in very special circumstances, everybody has rights. For example, they have a right to privacy, to be educated and to vote. They have a right to safety and protection, to freedom from abuse, to marry and to have a family life. They have a right to have their own views and beliefs and to be able to say how they feel. They also have a right to refuse any help that is offered them. Denying people their rights makes them feel that they don't count, that they are worthless.

Respecting people's rights in the way you work with them shows that you value them. For example, by respecting your colleagues' and service users' rights to hold opinions that are different from yours and to feel free to express themselves will make them feel important and well-regarded.

Giving choices

Being able to make choices is a right that no-one should be denied. Sometimes we need help in making choices, for example if we don't have enough information about what to do in a difficult situation. Being able to make our own choices makes us feel good about ourselves and in control of our lives. Not being able to make choices when we want to and are able to can be frustrating and cause us to lose our individuality.

Encouraging people you work with to make choices and respecting the choices they make, for example about when to get up and go to bed, what to wear, what and when to eat, what to do and when to do it, shows you value them and want them to feel good and in control.

Respecting privacy

We have a right to have our privacy respected, for example in matters of personal hygiene, relationships, letters and telephone calls and in our financial affairs. Except in exceptional circumstances, no-one should interfere with what we want to be kept private. If someone invades our privacy we can lose trust in them and confidence in ourselves.

Respecting people's right to privacy in the way that you work with them shows you value them. For example, respect the closed door – it could mean that a private meeting or telephone conversation is taking place, or that someone is using the toilet or is having a bath. A letter, bank statement or pension book is private unless you have been given permission to read it; and two people locked in quiet conversation means that a private discussion may be taking place and you may not be welcome to join in.

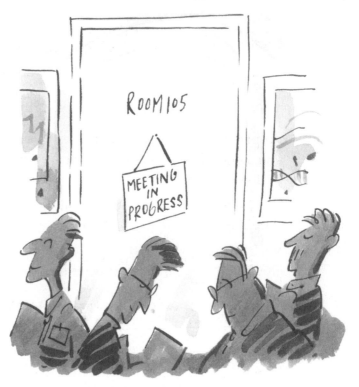

It is important to respect other people's privacy

Encouraging independence

Becoming independent is a normal part of human development. Staying as independent as possible is important because it means being able to do what we want, when we want. It means being responsible for ourselves, staying in control and living the life we want to live, being confident and having a feeling of self-worth.

Helping people to stay independent in the way that you work with them shows that you value them. It means respecting whatever independence they already have and encouraging them to be as responsible for themselves as they can, for example in managing their workload and money, in dealing with their relationships, in getting around and in maintaining their own personal hygiene and appearance.

Preserving dignity

Dignity is about self-respect and being proud of ourselves. We feel dignified when, for example, we behave, dress or do our job in the ways that we feel are right and proper and that we are comfortable with. If our dignity is taken away, we can feel cheapened and degraded and we lose our pride.

Respecting people's dignity in the way that you work with them shows you value them. If a colleague or service user has a preference for a way of doing things or of presenting themselves to others, you should respect that preference and not force your ways and ideas on to them. You should always help others to feel proud of themselves.

Working in partnership

Most of our working lives are spent with other people, for example with service users and their families and friends, with colleagues and representatives from other organisations. We work in partnership with these people and each person has a different role to play in the partnership.

For a working partnership to be successful, you have to show your partners that you value what they bring to the partnership, for example their individuality, knowledge and experience.

DEVELOP GOOD WORK PRACTICE 1.1.1

ACTIVITY 1

CASE STUDY: Emma

Emma has been a wheelchair user since she was a child, although she can walk short distances with the aid of crutches. Apart from you, she is supported by a general practitioner (GP), a social worker and a physiotherapist. She is a member of the Labour Party, a vegetarian and has lately become interested in doing some voluntary work.

Complete the table to show how you would use the care values and the importance of using the care values in your work with Emma.

Care value	How you would use the care values in your work with Emma	Why you should use the care values in your work with Emma
Showing respect		
Recognising individuality		
Giving choices		
Respecting privacy		
Encouraging independence		
Preserving dignity		
Working in partnership		

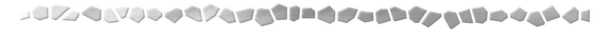

Prejudice

We all tend to judge people before we know them properly. We pre-judge them.

Prejudices are the ideas and beliefs we have about the people we pre-judge. They are usually negative thoughts that are based on people's:

- age
- sex
- appearance, including their size and skin colour
- inability to do certain things (disability)
- job and social class
- religion
- politics.

Your prejudices must never be allowed to influence the way that you do your work. If, for example, you are prejudiced against someone because of the colour of their skin, their age or their religion and you show your negative thoughts in the way you work with them, you will be behaving in a discriminatory way.

Equal opportunities

Discriminatory behaviour flies in the face of the care values that you have just learned about. People working in the caring services are duty-bound to work with people in a way that does not discriminate. Instead, their work must be based on equal opportunities. This means that caring organisations must ensure that each of its employees and service users, regardless of their age, sex, colour, abilities, religion and so on, is treated fairly and in keeping with their needs.

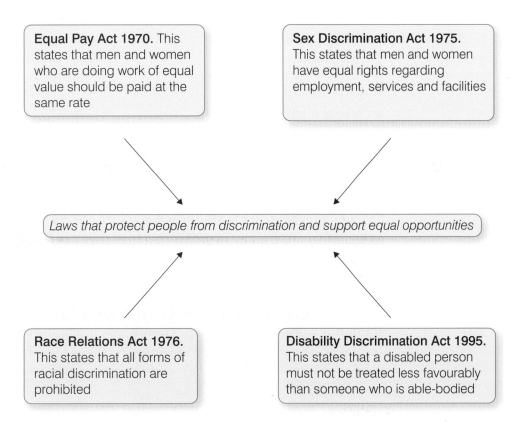

Equal Pay Act 1970. This states that men and women who are doing work of equal value should be paid at the same rate

Sex Discrimination Act 1975. This states that men and women have equal rights regarding employment, services and facilities

Laws that protect people from discrimination and support equal opportunities

Race Relations Act 1976. This states that all forms of racial discrimination are prohibited

Disability Discrimination Act 1995. This states that a disabled person must not be treated less favourably than someone who is able-bodied

ACTIVITY 2

Make notes on:

- why you think people might be prejudiced against your service users
- how you think you can use equal opportunities in your work with service users.

Discuss your thoughts with your supervisor.

1.2 RELATIONSHIPS AT WORK

Relationships with service users

Think about the people you know and with whom you have relationships. If you were to make a list of the relationships you have, you might include:

- family relationships
- friendships
- sexual relationships
- working relationships.

Good relationships are very important. Family, friends, sexual partners and work colleagues, in one way or another, offer each other companionship, advice, support, a sense of belonging and the opportunity to share experiences such as a day out shopping or an evening at the pub. As a result of having good relationships with people, we feel valued and cared for.

Because <u>care workers</u> work with service users, the relationship between them is a working relationship. Friendships might form; and there are instances where care workers and service users have fallen in love and settled down together. But generally speaking, because care workers are employed to work with service users, the relationship that develops between them has to be different from a friendship, family or sexual relationship.

CASE STUDY: **Lena and Molly**

Lena and Molly have been friends for years. They have been there for each other through thick and thin. Until recently, that is, when Molly heard on the grapevine that Lena has been talking about her behind her back, criticising her and spreading rumours about her that are hurtful and untrue.

Friendships can go sour. Do you think that this sort of behaviour would be acceptable if Lena was Molly's care worker? No, it wouldn't. Lena's behaviour doesn't show respect for Molly and it disregards the privacy of the relationship they had shared.

CASE STUDY: **Tom and Danny**

Danny has a sight impairment and his dad Tom has always considered himself to be Danny's 'eyes'. Lately, Danny's vision has become worse and Tom now feels he must now do everything for him, including bathing and feeding him and choosing his clothes for him.

Tom is a good dad – he has always been supportive of Danny and Danny will have benefited from his help over the years. But should a care worker behave in the way that Tom has started doing? No, because his behaviour doesn't respect Danny's privacy, nor does it encourage him to be independent and make choices. Friends and relatives, out of the goodness of their hearts or out of duty, can sometimes take on too much.

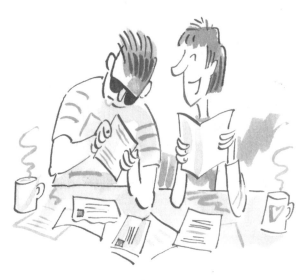

A professional relationship must be maintained between a care worker and a service user

CASE STUDY: *Carla and Jack*

Carla is very supportive of her neighbour Jack, who has multiple sclerosis. Recently Jack asked her if she would help him have a bath. Because they have been such good friends for a long time, Carla agreed to help and one thing led to another …

This is the stuff that movies are made from! But do you think that having a sexual relationship with a service user is appropriate behaviour for a paid care worker? No, it isn't. Sexual relationships bring people very close emotionally and emotions can get in the way of giving good, professional care.

Relationships between friends, family members and sexual partners can lack one or other of the care values. As a care worker your priority is to develop a working relationship with your service users in which you use all the care values in your work. The next section will look at the responsibilities and limits of a working relationship.

CHECK YOUR UNDERSTANDING

 1.2.1

ACTIVITY 3

Make a list of the differences between your relationships with service users, friends and members of your family.

Service users	Family members	Friends

The responsibilities and limits of a worker relationship

You wouldn't be employed as a care worker if you weren't a friendly person. But your priority is to develop working relationships with your service users that, while friendly, avoid the drawbacks of other types of relationship you have with people in your personal life.

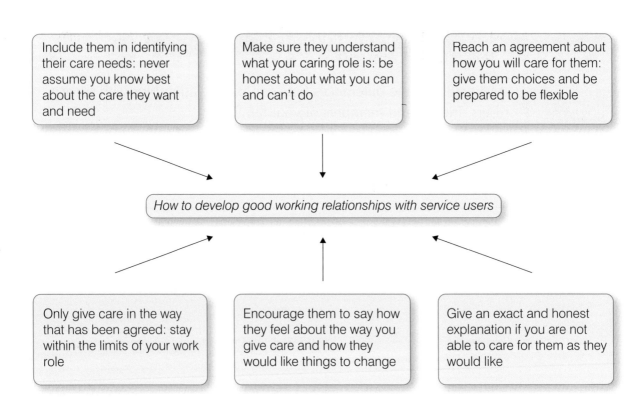

Include them in identifying their care needs: never assume you know best about the care they want and need

Make sure they understand what your caring role is: be honest about what you can and can't do

Reach an agreement about how you will care for them: give them choices and be prepared to be flexible

How to develop good working relationships with service users

Only give care in the way that has been agreed: stay within the limits of your work role

Encourage them to say how they feel about the way you give care and how they would like things to change

Give an exact and honest explanation if you are not able to care for them as they would like

CHECK YOUR UNDERSTANDING

 1.2.2

ACTIVITY 4

CASE STUDY: *Abdul*

Abdul has recently moved into The Beeches Residential Home. Bob, a care worker, has told Abdul not to worry, he won't have to say a word because Bob knows exactly what his service users are thinking and he'll take care of everything for Abdul in the way that he knows best. And if Abdul wants anything doing at any time of the day or night, he'll be there to do it for him.

Make a list of the ways that Bob's behaviour is unacceptable in terms of his relationship with Abdul.

_____

_____

_____

_____

_____

_____

_____

_____

_____

_____

_____

Reporting your worries

In addition to being responsible for developing good working relationships with your service users, you are also responsible for reporting anything you see at work that worries you.

Abuse of service users is very worrying indeed (see Chapter 9). Abuse is hurting or bullying someone physically, sexually, emotionally or financially. It can take place wherever care is given, but if you use the care values in your work with service users and:

- respect them and their need for dignity
- show them that you value them as individuals

- protect their rights and give them choices
- encourage them to be independent
- work with them as equal partners

you can be confident that your behaviour will not be abusive in any way.

The sorts of things that should concern you and which could be the result of abuse of service users include:

- unusual injuries, e.g. bruises, cuts, burns, bleeding
- changes in behaviour, e.g. crying, depression, fear, wanting to be alone and inappropriate or unusual sexual behaviour
- changes in condition, e.g. poor hygiene, loss of appetite and weight
- loss of money or other personal belongings

There are always reasons why people behave abusively. Service users, perhaps because they have been discriminated against or are frightened, stressed or are using drugs, can behave as abusively as anybody else. If you are worried that a service user is being abused or if you see anybody behaving in an abusive way, then it is your responsibility to report your concerns without delay.

The purpose of reporting abuse is to protect people, including care workers, from abusive behaviour. Tell your supervisor how you feel or what you have seen. Their experience will enable them to deal with the situation. They will also be able to talk you through your concerns and offer guidance as to how you could behave in similar situations in the future.

Make enquiries about any training that may be available to you on dealing with abusive, challenging behaviour.

1.2.3

What do you think?

ACTIVITY 5

You have started work in a day care centre but are concerned because the toilet doors have no locks, there is never a choice of what to eat for lunch and a number of the care workers use language that is insulting to the service users.

Your feeling is that the care workers are being abusive to the service users.

Note down why you think that behaviour like this is abusive and what you should do about your concerns.

_____

_____

_____

_____

_____

_____

_____

_____

_____

_____

_____

_____

1.3 COMMUNICATION

Verbal and non-verbal communication

The ability to communicate is very important. It allows us to interact with other people and form relationships with them. And because care work goes hand-in-hand with the development of good relationships with service users, good communication is a skill that you need to develop.

We don't need to be able to talk, speak the same language, hear or see in order to communicate with each other. There are a variety of communication aids and techniques such as pictures, sign language, Braille and interpreters that can be used to help people communicate. For a communication to take place, what *is* needed are people who have thoughts, feelings or information to share with each other.

In situations where speech or verbal communication is possible, only about 10% of a communication is spoken. The other 90% is through body language or non-verbal communication.

However, verbal communication is very useful. If we speak clearly we can:

- let others know how we feel and what we want
- find out about things by asking questions
- pass on information and give directions.

To prove to yourself just how useful words are, try asking someone, *without speaking,* for a cup of tea! It's good to talk!

Body language (non-verbal communication) is perhaps more important than speech – it tells people how we truly feel, something that words on their own aren't very good at. And the appropriate use of body language when communicating with service users will show them that you respect them and value what they have to say. Body language takes a number of forms.

- **Facial expressions**, e.g. smiles, frowns, looks of amazement and disgust. Saying something with a smile on your face gives a totally different meaning from saying the same thing with a look of fear!

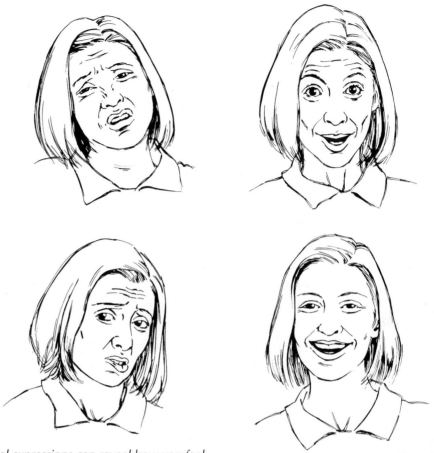

Facial expressions can reveal how you feel

- **Eye contact.** Appropriate use of eye contact lets a person know that you are interested in what they have to say and gazing into somebody's eyes can be a sign of a romantic attachment! But looking out of the window while they talk or staring at them for long periods will not help a communication along. You will look bored and may cause the speaker to become anxious.

- **Body posture and position.** If you slouch or turn away while someone is talking to you, you will look fed up and totally uninterested in the communication. Leaning slightly toward a person in an upright but comfortable position shows you are alert and giving them your full attention.

- **Body movements.** Tapping your foot or fingers while someone is talking to you is a sure sign that you are bored, perhaps in a hurry and don't want to listen. On the other hand, nodding your head shows that you understand what the other person is saying and moving your hands gives expression to what you are saying.

- **Dress.** The way you dress says a great deal about you. It tells people who you are, what your job is, and whether you have power or influence over them. So be aware of the effect you can have on people if, for example, you wear a uniform.
- **Touch and closeness.** Touching and being physically close to someone can be a useful way of showing your concern for them or that you are pleased to see them. But beware – you must be guided by whether the other person wants to be touched or not and by the 'personal space' they need to surround themselves with.

Finally, how a person says their words can speak volumes about how they feel. When people are feeling sad or depressed, they tend to speak quietly, slowly, on a low note and without much variation in their tone of voice. But when they are excited or anxious they speak more loudly and quickly, with ups and downs in their tone of voice.

CHECK YOUR UNDERSTANDING 1.3.1

ACTIVITY 6

Observe and make a note of the verbal and non-verbal methods of communication your colleagues and service users use when communicating with each other. Discuss your observations with your supervisor and explain why these methods were used.

_____

_____

_____

_____

_____

1.4 CONFIDENTIALITY

The importance of confidentiality

<u>Confidentiality</u> is to do with privacy and with being discreet.

Privacy is a care value that you must use in your work with service users. As you read earlier, except in special circumstances everybody has a right to have their privacy respected, both in their personal lives and in their affairs with other people and organisations.

Being discreet means being careful about the kind of information you pass on and who you pass it to. The Data Protection Act and your workplace policies and procedures tell you what information can be passed on and to whom.

In order to carry out your role as a care worker, you will have been made aware of a great deal of very personal information about your service users.

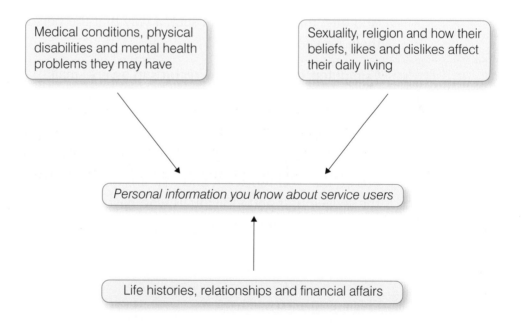

Service users may feel that this sort of information is very private and it may have been difficult for them to reveal it to you.

How do you think you would feel if details about your personal life became common knowledge? You might feel distressed and angry; and you would lose trust in the individual who disregarded your privacy. Imagine how a vulnerable service user would feel in the same position. You are therefore privileged to have been given such personal information and it is your responsibility to safeguard it within the organisation you work for. By demonstrating your ability to maintain the confidentiality of service users personal information, you will prove your trustworthiness.

Personal information about service users is recorded in a number of ways, including in their:

- care plans and case notes
- medical records
- Medicines Administration Records
- observation charts.

All records should be accurate, legible (readable), clear, to the point and only contain information that is useful and relevant and can be shared. And they must be stored in such a way that the personal details within them remain confidential.

Computers can store many records in a very small space. The advantage of storing records in computers is that you can control who sees them by the use of computer passwords. Confidentiality of written records is maintained by locking them in filing cabinets. If you remove a service user's record from its safe storage place you must take great care to ensure that you replace it and that it is not seen by anybody other than the service user and individuals who have been given permission to see it, such as members of the care team.

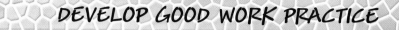

DEVELOP GOOD WORK PRACTICE 1.4.1

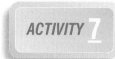

ACTIVITY 7 Find out from your colleagues how and why confidentiality is maintained in your workplace. Complete the table to demonstrate your understanding.

How confidentiality is maintained at work	Why confidentiality is maintained at work

The limits of confidentiality

There may be some occasions when you will need to 'break' confidentiality. What this means is that 'need-to-know' information about a service user can be passed on without his or her permission. However, except in exceptional circumstances, the service user must be told exactly what information has been passed on (disclosed) as soon as possible.

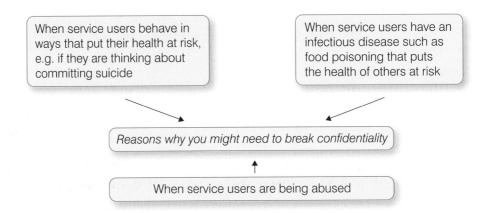

When service users behave in ways that put their health at risk, e.g. if they are thinking about committing suicide

When service users have an infectious disease such as food poisoning that puts the health of others at risk

Reasons why you might need to break confidentiality

When service users are being abused

Because of the possibility of needing to break confidentiality, if a service user asks you to keep a secret, you should hear what it is before you make any promises. And if you feel that you need to pass on what they tell you, you should reassure them that you are doing so in their best interests and that you will only tell people who are there to help.

DEVELOP GOOD WORK PRACTICE

 1.4.2

ACTIVITY 8

Talk to your supervisor about who you can disclose information to and under what circumstances.

Who I can disclose information to	Circumstances when I should disclose information

The importance of checking people's identity

Family members and friends want to be given news about service users. However, you may only give them information with the service user's permission. It may be, for example, that service users don't want family and friends to know why or how they are receiving care.

You may receive enquiries about service users from people on the telephone. But you must not disclose anything about a service user unless you:

- recognise the caller's voice
- have confirmed their identity (you could ask for their phone number, check it out and ring them back)
- have permission to give out information, for example to family and friends or to colleagues who need information in order to do their job.

If a visitor arrives at your workplace making enquiries about a service user, before you let them in you should:

- confirm their identity (they may have an official ID card or a driving licence)
- confirm with your supervisor that they have a right to visit
- check with the service user that they wish to see the visitor.

The same rules apply to people who ask about your colleagues. Always:

- confirm their identity
- if it's a visitor, check whether your colleague wishes to see them
- never give out any information unless you have your colleague's consent to do so.

CHECK YOUR UNDERSTANDING 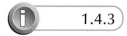 1.4.3

ACTIVITY 9

1 A young man arrives at your workplace wanting to know how his aunty, a resident with you, is getting on. Jot down what you should do.

_____

_____

_____

_____

2 You answer the phone and the caller asks you for your manager's home phone number. Jot down what you should do.

_____

_____

_____

_____

Discuss your responses with your supervisor.

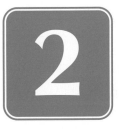

Understanding your workplace and your role as worker

All workplaces have aims or goals and the role of everyone associated with a workplace is to work together to achieve those goals. Workplaces also have principles (values or beliefs) about how their goals should be achieved. Workplaces whose goal is to deliver care services believe that the principles of care set the standards for how people should work together.

For care workers to deliver care in the way that is required of them they need to have a knowledge and understanding of their employer's aims and values. This chapter will help you identify your employer's aims and values and understand how they influence the way you do your job. It also builds on what you learned in Chapter 1 about the importance of developing good working relationships with service users.

Successful completion of the activities in this chapter will enable you to demonstrate your understanding of the Induction Standard *Understand the organisation and role of the worker*. It will also give you an opportunity to develop evidence for key skills unit Communication at level 1.

What is covered in this chapter?

This chapter contributes to the knowledge and understanding you need for the following NVQ Care units:

O1   : Foster people's equality, diversity and rights

CU1 : Promote, monitor and maintain health, safety and security in the workplace

CU3 : Monitor and maintain the cleanliness of environments

CU5 : Receive, transmit, store and retrieve information

CU10: Contribute to the effectiveness of work teams

W2   : Contribute to the ongoing support of clients and others significant to them

W8   : Enable individuals to maintain contact in potentially isolating situations

Z1   : Contribute to the protection of individuals from abuse

Z7   : Contribute to the movement and handling of clients to maximise their physical comfort

2.1 WORKPLACE POLICIES AND PROCEDURES

A policy is an official document that gives information about what must be done within a particular workplace, e.g. residential home, service user's own home. It sets out the workplace's responsibilities by describing the standards that workers have to use in their work. A workplace will have a number of policies, each one ensuring that one or more different laws are obeyed.

For example, a workplace's Health and Safety Policy spells out its responsibilities in making sure that health and safety laws and regulations are obeyed. It contains information about the standards of safe and healthy working that workers have to follow in their work.

A procedure is a document that explains to workers how they should do their jobs, i.e. it translates or interprets policies into working methods. Procedures also explain how to do a job in such a way that workers use the workplace's values or principles in getting the job done.

For example, a workplace's Health and Safety Policy will include information about the standards of safe and healthy working to be followed when dealing with hazardous substances like kitchen cleaning materials and body waste. A procedure will explain to you exactly how to work with, for example, bleach, blood and urine. By following the written procedure, you can be confident that you are obeying the law and so protecting the health and safety of everyone concerned. Equally importantly, you will be applying your workplace's principles of care.

It is very important to follow your workplace's policies and procedures for the following reasons:

- to obey the law – if a workplace is found to be disobeying the law, it can be closed down
- to safeguard the health and safety of everyone within the workplace
- to encourage and maintain good working practices
- to maintain a reputation as a trustworthy and respectable service provider – service users and service providers, including workers like yourself, all benefit from being associated with a workplace that has a good reputation.

CHECK YOUR UNDERSTANDING

 2.1.1

ACTIVITY 10

One of your service users has had a nose bleed and you have been asked to mop up the blood. Note down:

1 the type of workplace document that would tell you how to mop up the blood

_____

2 the type of workplace document that would contain information about standards of safe and healthy working that you should follow in dealing with body fluids like blood

_____

3 why you must follow the instructions given in these documents.

_____

_____

Policies and procedures at your workplace

Ignorance is no excuse in the eyes of the law. A judge wouldn't let you off a fine because you didn't know you had to tax and insure your car. It is your responsibility to know what the law is. In the same way, it is your responsibility to know the policies and procedures that affect what and how you do your job.

Your contract of employment will tell you that you have to work to policies and procedures. Be aware that you can be held responsible if your actions, omissions (what you don't do but should), errors or blunders result in things going wrong at work.

Where are your workplace policies and procedures stored? They are usually kept in files or folders in a central site office. You need to ask your supervisor exactly where they can be found, study the ones that affect you, and then be certain to use them in your work.

DEVELOP GOOD WORK PRACTICE 2.1.2

ACTIVITY 11

Find out and make a note of where your workplace policies and procedures are stored.

_____

_____

_____

2.2 POLICIES AND PROCEDURES RELATING TO YOUR JOB ROLE

There are a number of laws and regulations that determine the policies and procedures for workplaces providing care services. They include:

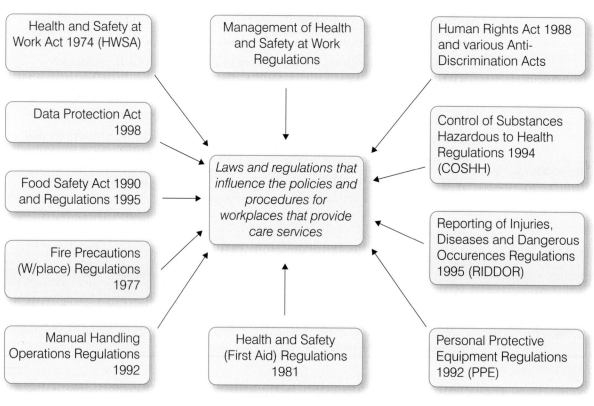

Health and Safety at Work Act 1974 (HWSA)

Management of Health and Safety at Work Regulations

Human Rights Act 1988 and various Anti-Discrimination Acts

Data Protection Act 1998

Control of Substances Hazardous to Health Regulations 1994 (COSHH)

Food Safety Act 1990 and Regulations 1995

Laws and regulations that influence the policies and procedures for workplaces that provide care services

Reporting of Injuries, Diseases and Dangerous Occurences Regulations 1995 (RIDDOR)

Fire Precautions (W/place) Regulations 1977

Manual Handling Operations Regulations 1992

Health and Safety (First Aid) Regulations 1981

Personal Protective Equipment Regulations 1992 (PPE)

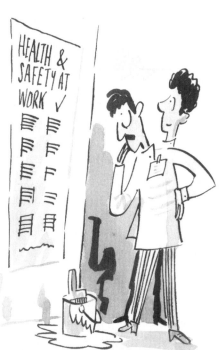

It is important to be aware of the health and safety laws and regulations

Workplace policies and procedures influenced by these laws and regulations that you should know about include:

Policies and procedures	What the policies and procedures cover
Health and safety	Everyone's responsibilities in helping keep the workplace free from health and safety risks Everyone's rights to information and training about health and safety issues
Responding to abuse	What to do when there is a risk of abuse, what to do after an abusive incident and how to report and record abuse Everyone's rights to support and to training on recognising and dealing with abuse
Confidentiality and disclosure of information	What information must be kept confidential, where it should be stored, who it may be disclosed (made known) to and why
Control of exposure to hazardous waste	Whether waste is hazardous or not, health and safety risks of working with hazardous waste, how to protect against risks, how to dispose of waste safely and what to do if there is an accident involving hazardous waste
Fire safety	What to do to prevent fire and the emergency action to take if there is a fire
Hygiene and food safety	Safe and hygienic food storage, preparation, cooking and serving in order to protect against food poisoning
Moving and handling	The need to assess (check) moving and handling risks. They also describe safe ways to move and handle loads, including service users
Dealing with accidents and emergencies	The need to have named, qualified first-aiders in the workplace, how to send for the emergency health services and how to record accidents and injuries What should be in the first aid box and who is responsible for maintaining the first aid box. Also about ensuring training in first aid
Infection control	Precautions to be taken when working with service users who have infectious diseases. Also about whether infections need to be reported and who to
Record keeping and access to files	Everyone's responsibilities to report, record and file information as requested by the supervisor or manager

What do you think?   2.2.1

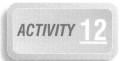

ACTIVITY 12

Note down three of your work tasks. For each one, write down the type of policy and procedures that you think are important for you to know about so that you can work properly and safely.

Work task	Policies and procedures

Discuss what you have written down with your supervisor.

2.2 YOUR JOB ROLE

You as an employee

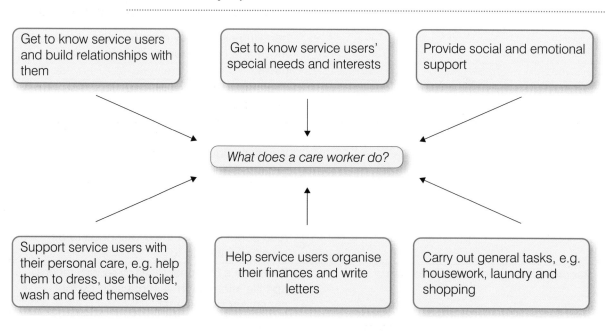

Get to know service users and build relationships with them

Get to know service users' special needs and interests

Provide social and emotional support

What does a care worker do?

Support service users with their personal care, e.g. help them to dress, use the toilet, wash and feed themselves

Help service users organise their finances and write letters

Carry out general tasks, e.g. housework, laundry and shopping

Your job may involve doing these things and many more. When you were interviewed for your job you were told what the job involved. Your contract of employment describes in writing what you are expected to do. But whatever your various tasks are, the most important thing to bear in mind is that you should work with your service users, not for them.

By working with service users, you will be helping your workplace to achieve its aim or goal of providing care. Most workplaces that provide care services sum up their aims in their Mission Statements and/or Charters of Care. Mission Statements and Charters of Care also tell you what a workplace's principles or values are by saying how they provide the service. An example of a mission statement that describes a workplace's aim and values is:

> Our aim is to work with service users in providing them with care that encourages them to be independent and to make choices and that respects their individuality, privacy and dignity.

DEVELOP GOOD WORK PRACTICE 2.3.1

ACTIVITY 13

Note down three of your work tasks and briefly describe how you use the principles of care in carrying out each task.

Work task	Principles of care used when carrying out each task

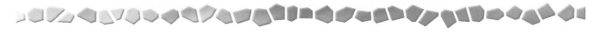

Compare what you have written with your workplace's aims and values. Your supervisor will be able to tell you what they are or there may be a workplace mission statement or care charter. Briefly describe how what you do helps your workplace to achieve its aims and values.

You as a team player

When you applied for your job, you were probably asked how you got on with others. This is because care workers need to be interested in and enjoy being with people. They also need to be able to build relationships with people from different walks of life. Care work itself is carried out by teams of people so care workers also need to develop good teamwork skills.

There will be very few occasions when you find yourself working alone. First and foremost, you will be working with your service users, their family, carers and friends. You will also be part of a work team. Work teams in the caring services each have their own specific functions and include:

- the caretaking team, e.g. gardeners, odd-job people
- the domestic team, e.g. cleaners, kitchen and laundry staff
- the health care team, e.g. health care assistants, nurses, doctors, physiotherapists
- the management and administration team
- the social care team, e.g. porters, care workers, social workers, occupational therapists.

Each team is as important as the next and one team can't function without the contribution of others. Care workers communicate with many of these teams. For example, the kitchen team can't do its job without instructions from care workers about service users' dietary needs; and the health care team needs care workers to keep them informed about service users' state of health.

It is important that you know what team members' job roles and responsibilities are. There is little point telling admin staff that Mrs J

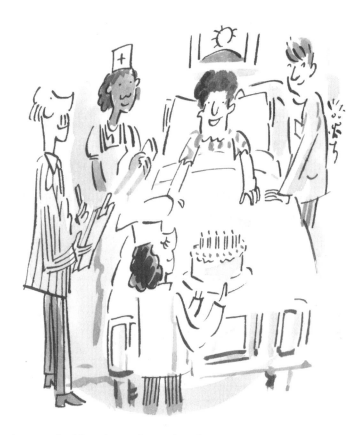

Each person has a valuable role to play within the care team

doesn't like cheese sandwiches any more. It is only necessary to give this information to colleagues who work directly with Mrs J, such as other members of the care team and the kitchen staff. You can find out about job roles and responsibilities by talking with colleagues and by reading job descriptions.

It isn't only workers who have roles and responsibilities. Your service users, their family, carers and friends have roles and responsibilities in working with you. For example they should:

- be honest and open when expressing their feelings about the care that you are giving
- be supportive and considerate of you as you carry out your caring role.

CHECK YOUR UNDERSTANDING

 2.3.2

ACTIVITY 14

Make a list of the people you work with in supporting one of your service users. Hopefully your list will include the service user! Use initials only to maintain confidentiality. Alongside their initials, jot down each person's main role and responsibility. Discuss what you have written with your supervisor to check that your understanding is correct.

People I work with   Their main roles and responsibilities

_____   _____

_____   _____

_____   _____

_____   _____

_____   _____

_____   _____

_____   _____

_____   _____

_____   _____

Getting help to do your job

We all need information, advice and support from time to time if we are to enjoy our jobs, perform them well and be satisfied in what we do.

You might want to know more about the organisation you work for, e.g. if you want to move up the career ladder but don't know what other jobs are available and what qualifications you need to be able to do them. You might want advice about an issue at work that you don't know how to deal with, e.g. how to challenge a colleague whom you feel is a bully. Or you might want guidance and support, e.g. if there are problems at home and you're concerned that they could affect your work.

Sources of information, advice and support available to you about your workplace include:

- your colleagues, your supervisor and your manager
- your workplace charters and policies
- your Trade Union representative
- professional organisations such as the Care Homes Association
- the Care Standards Commission.

Sources of information, advice and guidance available to you about work roles include:

- your colleagues, your supervisor and your manager
- your workplace policies and procedures
- official codes of practice and standards, e.g. TOPSS standards
- your Trade Union representative
- job descriptions and personal specifications
- your workplace training officer and NVQ assessor
- your mentor or workplace learning representative/support worker
- care publications, e.g. journals, magazines, books
- professional organisations such as the Care Homes Association
- the Care Standards Commission.

ACTIVITY 15

CASE STUDY: **Lisa**

Lisa has been a part-time assistant in the kitchen where you work for a number of years. She is thinking about working full-time as a cook or care worker. She doesn't know very much about the organisation, nor about the roles of a cook or care worker.

Complete the table with sources of information, advice and support that you think would help Lisa make a decision about her future.

Sources of information, advice and support about your workplace	Sources of information, advice and support about the role of a cook	Sources of information, advice and support about the role of a care worker

You and your supervisor

Your supervisor is there to help you develop and improve your workplace skills and relationships. You should feel able to approach your supervisor for advice and guidance on anything that concerns you. By talking things through with your supervisor, listening to what they say and acting on what they tell you, you will become a skilled and valued team member and employee. More importantly, you will earn the respect, admiration and appreciation of your service users.

There are two types of supervision: formal and informal.

Formal supervision happens on a planned basis. Appraisal is an example of formal supervision. You will be asked to attend appraisal meetings at times laid down in your workplace's policy on supervision, e.g. every three or six months.

Appraisal is an opportunity for you and your supervisor to discuss how you are doing at work, to talk about your work goals and ambitions, and to agree an action plan that will help you achieve both your ambitions and the goals that your employer has for you. You will be given a date for your appraisal and an opportunity to prepare for it. It will take place in privacy.

Informal supervision is on-going. It takes place 'on the job', i.e. as you are working and when your skills and relationships can be observed.

Informal supervision happens all the time and takes the form of discussions with, for instance, colleagues, supervisors and NVQ assessors who know what your goals and ambitions are and who want you to succeed. They also know the workplace goals and can give you advice and support about how you can improve your performance.

DEVELOP GOOD WORK PRACTICE 2.3.4

ACTIVITY 16

Note down:

- the name of your supervisor: _____
- when you will be supervised: _____
- where you will be supervised: _____
- how you will be supervised: _____
  _____
- why you will be supervised: _____

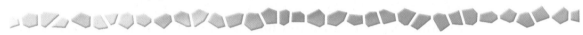

Working with service users' family and carers

Family, carers and service users are very important to each other. They need to be loved and valued by each other; they need to be able to give love and show how much they appreciate each other; and they need the security of continuing to be in a relationship with each other. For these reasons it is extremely important to include family and carers in service users' day-to-day lives.

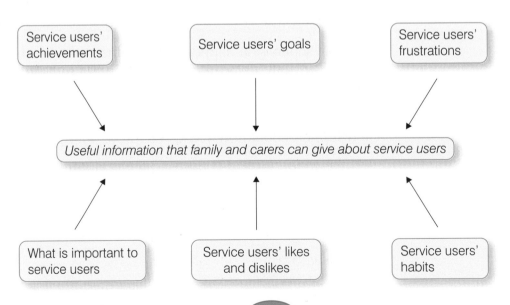

In addition to meeting your service users' need for love, self-esteem and security, family and carers can help you in your work by giving you information that your service users might not think to tell you.

Snippets of information like these help you get to know service users, help you build relationships with them, make you aware of their special needs and interests and guide you in giving them social and emotional support. Knowing such things ensures that you care for them as individuals with their own identity.

Involving family and carers in your care team and developing relationships with them also helps guard service users against neglect or abuse. Open, trusting relationships in which family, carers and care workers can voice their concerns will spot and prevent behaviour that may be abusive or neglectful.

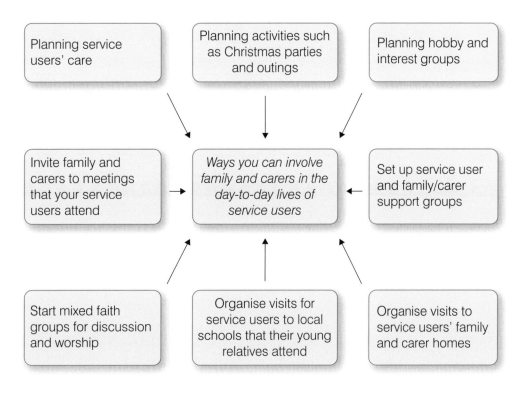

You could also talk with your supervisor or manager about ensuring that your workplace has an 'open-door' policy, i.e. family and carers are able to talk to the care team at any time.

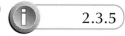

2.3.5

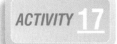

Write down three examples of how your workplace involves families and carers in the day-to-day lives of your service users. How does this involvement benefit service users, families, carers, you and your colleagues?

How families and carers are involved in service users' day-to-day lives	How the involvement of families and carers benefits everyone

3 Understanding the experiences and particular needs of service user groups

In this chapter you will learn about the different <u>service user groups</u> that care workers work with, the different needs that different service user groups have and the ways in which they can be supported. You will also build on your learning about the principles of care, your workplace's policies and procedures and your role as a worker.

Successful completion of the activities in this chapter will enable you to demonstrate your understanding of the Induction Standard *Understand the experiences and the particular needs of the service user groups*. It will also give you an opportunity to develop evidence for key skills unit Communication at level 1.

What is covered in this chapter?

This chapter contributes to the knowledge and understanding you need for the following NVQ Care units:

O1   : Foster people's equality, diversity and rights
CL1   : Promote effective communication and relationships
CL2   : Promote communication with individuals where there are communication differences
CL5   : Promote communication with those who do not use a recognised language format
NC12 : Help clients to eat and drink
Z6   : Enable clients to maintain and improve their mobility through exercise and the use of mobility appliances

> Z8 : Support individuals when they are distressed
> Z9 : Enable clients to maintain their personal hygiene and appearance
> Z11 : Enable clients to access and use toilet facilities
> Z19 : Enable clients to achieve physical comfort

3.1 TYPES OF SERVICE USER GROUP

What do we mean by 'service user group'?

A 'service provider' is an organisation that provides people with services, e.g. transport, communications, gas, water, electricity and of course health and personal care, housing and benefits.

A 'service user' is an individual who uses a service provider because the services it provides meets their needs. If you own a mobile phone, before you bought it you probably researched all the different mobile phone service providers to find the one whose service best met your needs in the way of rental costs, number of free calls and so on.

The service users that we are interested in are those who use care service providers. As a care worker, you will be employed by a care service provider, which may be your Local Authority Social Services Department or a private care agency.

In your role as a care worker, you may have the opportunity to work with different types of service user or 'service user groups'.

Because the people within a service user group have similar needs, there are service providers that exist specifically for them. For example, there are health service providers for people with mental health problems, personal social care service providers for people who are elderly and support groups that provide a service for people who have lost a loved one.

Different service user groups also have needs in common. For example, people with learning difficulties and people who are elderly are both likely to have needs associated with disabilities, confusion and specific health conditions. For this reason, it is important that you develop an understanding of how to meet a variety of needs.

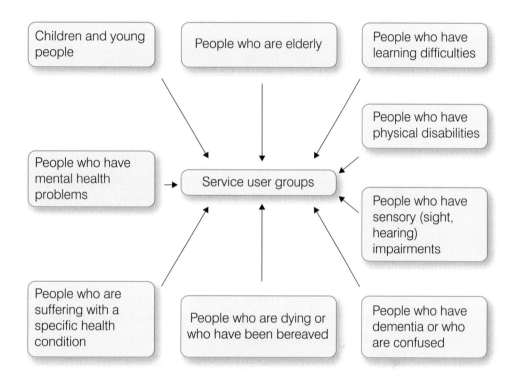

CHECK YOUR UNDERSTANDING   ⓘ   3.1.1

ACTIVITY 18

Note down which service user group(s) you work with:

_____

_____

Society's attitude to service users

If you look back at the examples of service user groups, you will see that each description began with 'People who …'. Describing service users in this way has regard to the values of care: respect is shown for the fact that they are, first and foremost, individuals; their characteristics as service users take second place.

CASE STUDY: *Jenny*

Jenny has had a stroke, is paralysed down her right side and is in a wheelchair. She is in her eighties and has difficulty hearing.

How would you describe Jenny? As a disabled, deaf, old woman? Hopefully you would say something along the lines of 'a lady who is elderly and who has a physical disability and a hearing impairment'. Describing her as a disabled, deaf, old woman makes her characteristics as a service user become the most important issue and we no longer see Jenny for herself.

Unfortunately many people in our society continue to judge others according to their special needs or characteristics. But what makes a person old or disabled?

Jenny wants to do a computer course so that she can e-mail her son in America. However, her nearest learning centre does not have wheelchair access.

How do you see Jenny now? Does it surprise you that a lady in her eighties is eager to learn new technologies? When do people become 'old'? 65? 80? What makes them 'old'? Wrinkles, grey hair, the clothes they wear? What does the term 'old' mean to you?

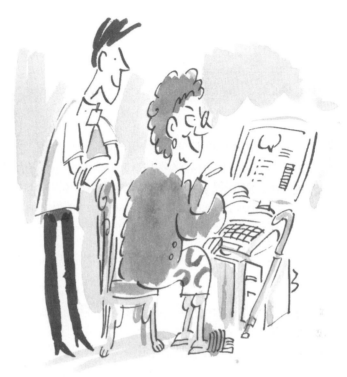

Modern technology can benefit everybody

What about the term 'disabled'? What makes a person disabled? What does the term mean to you? Jenny has a wheelchair so she can get around and go places – except to where the computer course is being held! Like lots of people in her situation, Jenny would probably tell you that she is not old or disabled – it is other people who describe her as old and it is the learning centre that is disabling her, holding her back her from what she wants to do.

So, not only does society make judgements about people with special needs or characteristics (see Chapter 1), as Jenny's case shows it also disables them, making it difficult and sometimes impossible for them to live their lives as they choose.

What do you think?

 3.1.2

ACTIVITY 19

CASE STUDIES: *Joe, Beverley and Nasser*

Joe, Beverley and Nasser all have mobility difficulties. Joe uses a walking frame but lives on a busy road where cars routinely park on the pavement. Beverley loves to go shopping for clothes but from her wheelchair she cannot reach the clothes hangers or see what is on the shelves above them. Nasser has difficulty getting on and off buses.

Make notes on changes that society could make so that life would be improved for:

1 Joe

_____

_____

_____

2 Beverley

_____

_____

_____

3 Nasser

_____

_____

_____

Discuss your ideas with your supervisor.

3.2 MEETING THE PARTICULAR NEEDS OF SERVICE USER GROUPS

A positive approach

It is very important that you care for your service users with a positive approach. This means:

- encouraging them to exercise (carry out) their rights, e.g. to make their own decisions and be as independent and responsible for themselves as they can
- respecting them as individuals, treating them fairly and not behaving in a discriminatory way
- ensuring that any information you are given about them remains confidential and is only shared with others who have a need to know.

> ### CASE STUDY: *Benjamin*
>
> *Benjamin, a West Indian, is becoming very old and frail. He doesn't seem to be eating properly and is showing signs of confusion. However, he is happy and enjoys the independence of living in his own home. His home care worker has told him that she is surprised his 'own people' aren't doing more for him and that she is going to talk to a friend of hers about getting him into a residential home.*

The care worker no doubt thinks that she is using a positive approach in her work with Benjamin. In reality this is not the case:

- her behaviour is discriminatory – she suggests that his 'own people' should be more responsible in the way they look after each other
- she is proposing to share information about him with someone who may not be authorised to know his personal details
- by interfering in where he lives, she is not encouraging him to make his own decisions and remain independent.

You may work with service users like Benjamin who concern you because you're not able to care for them in the way that you think would be best. In such situations it is quite a challenge to care with a positive approach. You will need to talk things through with your supervisor or manager. It could be that you are right in your concerns and that to care with a positive approach will require changing the way care is given. But it could also be that you need to think about your attitudes, ideas and beliefs and about how they influence the way you do your work.

DEVELOP GOOD WORK PRACTICE

(i) 3.2.1

ACTIVITY 20

Discuss with your supervisor how you could develop and use a positive approach in caring for your service users. Make notes on what you are told and briefly explain why it is important that you care in this way.

_____

_____

_____

_____

_____

_____

_____

_____

_____

_____

_____

_____

_____

_____

Service users who have personal care needs

Many service users need help in maintaining their personal hygiene. This may be because:

- they have had a stroke and are physically unable to care for themselves
- they have a learning difficulty and don't understand how to keep clean
- they don't have the money or resources, e.g. hot water, soap or clean clothing, needed to maintain their personal hygiene.

If you observe any changes in your service users' abilities to maintain their personal hygiene you should talk to your supervisor without delay.

Reasons why we should maintain good personal hygiene

Poor personal hygiene	Effects
Unwashed skin, particularly armpits, around the anus (back passage) and genitals (private parts)	Sweat and urine cause the skin to become smelly and sore; and dirty skin can be infected by itch mites (scabies)
Unwashed hair	Dirty, greasy hair is smelly and looks unpleasant
Unwashed feet	Dirty feet can be smelly and, if they're not dried properly, can be infected with athlete's foot/ringworm
Unclean mouth, teeth and dentures	Dirty teeth are at risk of decay and an unclean mouth, teeth and dentures look unpleasant and cause bad breath
Unclean nails and hands	Dirty nails are unattractive and can carry infections, e.g. when a person who has threadworms scratches their bottom, the threadworm eggs get stuck under their nails
Unclean clothes	Dirty clothes are smelly and feel and look unpleasant. They can also be a home to fleas and bed bugs

Poor personal hygiene is not only a health hazard, it also causes people to lose their pride in themselves. Service users are vulnerable to poor health and lack of self-respect. It is your responsibility to support them in maintaining their personal hygiene in ways that they are comfortable with.

Service users are assessed for the support they need in maintaining their personal cleanliness. Some may be confined to bed and need bed baths. Others need help with having a bath or a shower, with shaving, washing their hair and cleaning their teeth or dentures. You must follow workplace procedures and care plans in giving the agreed support and the way you care must always be in keeping with the care values.

Many of your service users will need help eating and drinking. This may be because:

- they are physically unable to feed themselves or see what they are doing
- they are confused and have forgotten how to eat and drink
- they are too upset to eat
- their dentures are uncomfortable.
- they are ill or on medication that reduces their appetite.

If you observe any changes in your service users' abilities to eat and drink you should talk to your supervisor without delay.

There are a number of aids such as two-handled cups and chunky cutlery that are designed to help service users eat and drink. There are also a number of ways to tempt them to eat, e.g. by giving choices of what, when and where to eat and who to eat with; by serving food in an attractive way; and by providing an enjoyable and relaxed atmosphere for eating in.

If your service users are not able to eat and drink independently, you will need to find out from them exactly what help they want and then be guided by them in giving that help. It is important when feeding service users that you help them at the speed with which they are happy, that you ensure they are comfortable, that you treat them as adults and maintain their pride and dignity and that they enjoy their mealtimes with you.

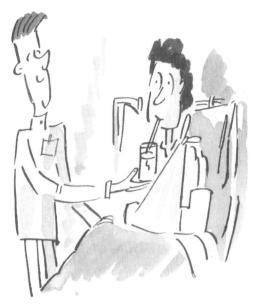

Make sure that meal times are comfortable and enjoyable for your service users

A number of service users will need support using the toilet. They may have a mobility problem that makes it difficult for them to walk to the toilet. This becomes a greater problem if they need to make frequent visits. They may suffer from 'urgency', which means they can't get to the toilet on time and they 'leak'. Leaking is a form of incontinence. If you observe any changes in your service users' abilities to use toilet facilities you should talk to your supervisor without delay.

It is very distressing for people when they realise they need support with using the toilet. It is also very embarrassing for them to ask for and to be given help. For this reason, you need to develop excellent communication skills that demonstrate that you are approachable, understanding and want to help them remain as independent as possible. And of course you need to have respect for the service users' dignity, privacy and need for confidentiality.

Your service users will have been assessed for the amount of help they need to use toilet facilities. Some may be able to get to the toilet or commode themselves or to use a bedpan, but others may need help. Some may need to use incontinence pads and others may have catheter bags. Your workplace procedures and service users' care plans will direct you in your work but, if you have any concerns, you should report these without delay to your supervisor.

Workplace procedures will also describe the precautions you should take in the handling and disposal (throwing away) of body waste (urine and faeces). Body waste can carry infectious diseases and must therefore be handled and disposed of safely and hygienically.

You may be asked to monitor service users' body waste. This means keeping a check on how often they use the toilet and what their urine and faeces look like. This is because both the number of times a person uses the toilet and the amount and appearance of their body waste can give clues about their state of health. Your workplace will have a procedures for collecting, checking and measuring body waste. It is very important that you follow these procedures at all times.

Many service users do not move about much and as a result they are at risk of getting pressure sores. A pressure sore is an area of the skin in which the blood supply has been cut off. As a result, the skin dies and breaks down. If you notice what might be a pressure sore developing on a service user, you should report your concerns without delay to your supervisor.

The most common places for pressure sores to occur are on the ears, back of the head, shoulder blades, elbows, buttocks, bottom of the back, heels and ankles. They are caused by:

- pressure on the skin from the hard parts of a bed or chair
- the skin being dragged as the person slips or slides down in bed
- friction on the skin caused by, for instance, wet incontinence pads, clothing and bedding.

Your service users will have been assessed for their risk of getting pressure sores and it is important that you follow procedures and care plans to prevent sores occurring. The best way is to encourage service users to keep moving but as that isn't always practicable there are a variety of aids that can be used. Aids include special mattresses, cushions and fleece pads that either reduce pressure on the skin or spread the pressure more evenly across the body. And of course keeping a service user dry is very important – bedding, clothing and pads should be changed immediately they become wet.

DEVELOP GOOD WORK PRACTICE   ⓘ   3.2.2

ACTIVITY 21

Look at the care plan of one of your service users and tick which of the following aspects of personal care they need support with:

- personal hygiene ☐
- eating and drinking ☐
- using the toilet ☐
- prevention of pressure sores ☐

Make brief notes on how the care plan tells you to support the service user.

_____

_____

_____

_____

_____

_____

_____

_____

_____

_____

_____

_____

_____

_____

_____

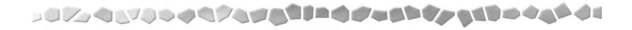

Dementia and confusion

We normally associate conditions like confusion and dementia, e.g. Alzheimer's disease, with service users who are elderly. However, they can occur in younger people and people in their mid-life. Suffering from dementia is distressing and working with someone who has dementia and is confused can be complicated. For example, communication becomes difficult because of the loss of short term memory (memory for recent events); they can be anxious, aggressive and abusive; and they can become quite childlike and dependent.

Dementia and confusion occur for a variety of reasons. Some service users benefit from medication that helps them remember things. Others can be helped by activities that stimulate the mind, e.g. puzzles and card games, or that encourage them to see the importance of their past, e.g. reminiscence therapy (talking about their younger days). You can support service users by helping them remember to take their medication; by helping them maintain a routine in their lives; by giving them time, being patient and showing them that you continue to value them; and by speaking clearly and simply yet without taking away their dignity.

CHECK YOUR UNDERSTANDING

 3.2.3

ACTIVITY 22

CASE STUDY: Kate

Kate has recently become a service user where you work. Your observations of her behaviour make you think that she has Alzheimer's disease.

Note down:

1 how Kate might be behaving to make you think she has Alzheimer's disease

_____

_____

_____

_____

_____

2 how you would care for Kate if she did have Alzheimer's disease.

_____

_____

_____

_____

_____

Discuss your notes with your supervisor to check your understandi

Death, dying and bereavement

People who are dying or who have been bereaved (lost a friend or loved one) are said to go through a number of stages as they adjust to their situation. Understanding people's feelings in these traumatic times will guide you in supporting them.

Stage 1: Denial
The person who is dying refuses to believe they are going to die
The bereaved person can't believe they have lost their loved one.

Stage 2: Anger
The person who is dying and the bereaved person are angry about their situation.

Stage 3: Depression
The person who is dying and the bereaved person are sad and full of despair.

Stage 4: Acceptance
The person who is dying accepts that death is coming. They become peaceful at last.
For the bereaved person, life at last begins to return to normal.

If your service user is dying, be there for them when they need you. Give them time to express how they feel and what they want to happen after they have passed away. Let them choose where to die and who they want around them. However, if what they want might not be appropriate for them and those closest to them, seek advice from your supervisor in helping them make these choices.

If you are helping to support bereaved family and friends, be there to listen to them and ensure that they have time and privacy to grieve. Check that they are given information about what needs to happen following the death; and inform them about sources of support and services that they might use.

Your own emotions will be running high at times like these. Don't be cautious about seeking support – you have a right to feel upset and distressed and your supervisor will want to help you.

CHECK YOUR UNDERSTANDING

 3.2.4

ACTIVITY 23

Talk with your supervisor about your role in caring for dying service users and in supporting their bereaved family and friends. Make a list of your responsibilities.

_____

_____

_____

_____

_____

_____

_____

Service users who experience specific conditions

You have by now come across a number of terms that describe specific conditions and their effects on service users. Specific conditions include:

- **Mobility problems.** This term describes the condition where a service user has difficulty moving around because of restricted use of his legs and feet
- **Pressure sores.** This term describes the condition that results from pressure or friction on the skin
- **Dementia.** This term describes the condition where a service user is confused and has a problem with, for example, short-term memory or communication.

Your service users may be experiencing one or a number of different conditions. It is important that you have an understanding of their conditions and their effects so that you can give appropriate help and support.

CHECK YOUR UNDERSTANDING

 3.2.5

ACTIVITY 24

Talk to your supervisor about the effects of two different conditions on service users and how you can support them.

Complete the table to show your understanding.

Condition	Effect of the condition on the service user	How you can support service users with these conditions

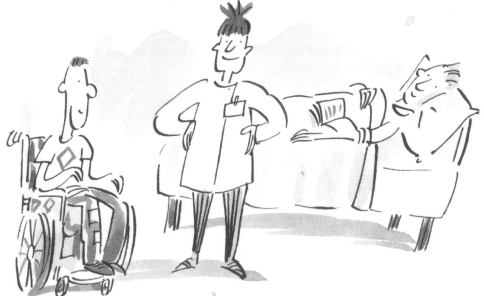

Your service users will have different conditions, which you must be aware of

Service users who have been prescribed medication

Many of your service users will have been prescribed medication by their GPs or hospital doctors.

Reasons why medication is prescribed	Examples of medications
To treat people and make them better	Antibiotics, which are prescribed to treat infections
To relieve symptoms and give relief	Painkillers, such as paracetamol
To prevent ill health	Aspirin, which is prescribed to reduce the risk of heart attack
To keep body functions as normal as possible	Insulin, which is prescribed for diabetics to keep their blood sugar levels within safe limits
To improve quality of life	Aricept (donepezil), which is prescribed to assist memory

If service users have been prescribed medication, it is very important that they take it. But unless you have been trained in medicines administration and are a 'designated person', you are not allowed to give medicines to your service users. Instead, your responsibility is to support and encourage them to take their medication, for example by:

- providing them with information about their medication
- making sure that the medicine is in a suitable form for them; for example, liquids are easier to swallow than tablets
- checking that they don't dislike the smell or taste of the medicine
- assisting them into a comfortable position that will make it easier for them to take their medicine
- checking that they have taken their medicine
- watching out for problems that might be linked to taking the medicine.

If you are concerned that your service users are experiencing problems to do with their medication or are not taking it as they should do, you should talk to your supervisor without delay.

CHECK YOUR UNDERSTANDING

 3.2.6

ACTIVITY 25

CASE STUDY: Michael

Michael has been taking tablets for his heart condition for a number of years. Lately he has developed a swallowing problem and you find a number of pills under the cushion of his chair. Write down what you should you do and why.

_____

_____

_____

_____

_____

_____

_____

_____

_____

_____

Service users who have unpredictable moods and behaviour

We all experience mood ups-and-downs and some of us can have a temper tantrum now and again even though we are normally quite well behaved! Emotional upsets like these can be caused by a number of factors, such as the way people treat us, illness, stress, worry and our frustrations with ourselves.

It is hardly surprising, then, that some service users have mood swings or behave in unpredictable (unexpected) ways. For example, people who are elderly may be anxious because they can no longer do what they used to do. People who have disabilities or learning difficulties may lose their temper because of the way people discriminate against them. In addition, many of the specific conditions experienced by service users, such as dementia and schizophrenia, have unexpected moods and behaviours as symptoms.

As a care worker, you need to know which service users have unpredictable moods and behaviours and how to respond to them. For example you need to know how to 'defuse' or calm abusive, aggressive and violent situations. Your workplace will have a procedure on how to deal with abuse, aggression and violence and you should make sure you follow it in your work.

Prevention, as always, is better than cure and preventing dangerous situations happening is preferable to having to deal with them. Watch out for any changes in your service users' moods and behaviour and report any concerns you have to your supervisor or manager.

DEVELOP GOOD WORK PRACTICE 3.2.7

ACTIVITY 26

Discuss with your supervisor and make notes on:
- what can trigger changes in mood and behaviour in your service users

_____

_____

_____

_____

_____

- the sorts of situations that can arise as a result of these changes

_____

_____

_____

_____

_____

- how you are expected to respond to these situations.

_____

_____

_____

_____

_____

Service users who neglect their own needs

You read earlier that we all have a right to freedom from abuse. Neglecting a service user by avoiding, overlooking or ignoring their care needs is a form of abuse. Unfortunately, service users are likely to neglect themselves, for example by:

- not taking their medication, eating and drinking properly, caring for their personal hygiene and appearance, looking after their own comfort
- not staying in touch with friends and family
- not saying what they want and how they feel.

There are many reasons why service users neglect themselves. They may be depressed; they may find it physically difficult to look after themselves; they may have forgotten how to care for themselves; or they may have simply lost interest in looking after themselves.

Once service users start to neglect themselves, their needs increase. It is your responsibility to watch out for any signs of self-neglect and to think about the reasons for the self-neglect. Discuss your concerns with your supervisor and suggest how to adapt the care you give to prevent a down-turn in their condition.

CHECK YOUR UNDERSTANDING

 3.2.8

ACTIVITY 27

CASE STUDY: Josie

Josie lives on her own. On your last visit, you noticed that her hair and clothes looked scruffy, there was a smell of urine about her, the house felt cold and she hadn't posted the birthday card she had written for her daughter. Your think Josie might be neglecting herself. Jot down how you would check this out and what you would do if your worry was confirmed.

Living with disabilities and impairments

Some service users need support in their day-to-day living if, for example, they have difficulty:

- moving around
- seeing
- hearing.

The most valuable support you can give is to check out how suitable their living environment is. If it is made safe and easy to move around in and to find things in, service users have a greater opportunity to be independent and to live their lives as they choose.

You can make living environments safe and easy to use for service users who have difficulty seeing and/or moving around by:
- having slopes instead of steps
- using floor coverings that are smooth, not slippery and not likely to cause trips
- arranging furniture so that it doesn't block passageways.

There are also numerous aids and adaptations such as wheelchairs, walking frames, stairlifts and grab rails that can make life easier.

You can also support service users who have a sight impairment by:
- making sure that they have their eyesight tested regularly and that their glasses are clean and worn properly
- making sure that their possessions are kept in the same, familiar places
- supporting them in their use of a sighted guide, cane or guide dog
- training to be a sighted guide yourself.

There are also aids and adaptations available to help people with a sight impairment, including magnifying glasses and newspapers and books in large print.

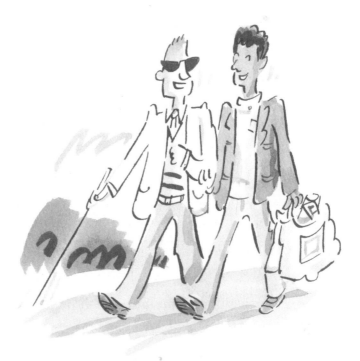

There are many ways to help a service user to be as independent as possible

You can support service users who have a hearing impairment by:

- making sure that their hearing is regularly checked and that their hearing aids work, are clean and are worn properly
- using communication techniques that meet their needs, e.g. speaking clearly, using sign language
- providing alternatives to doorbells, fire alarms or ringing telephones such as flashing lights and pieces of equipment that vibrate.

CHECK YOUR UNDERSTANDING

 3.2.9

ACTIVITY 28

Carry out a survey of your workplace and list the ways in which it makes life as easy as possible for:

1 service users who have a mobility problem

2 service users who have a sight impairment

3 service users who have a hearing impairment.

Discuss with your supervisor how life might be further improved for these service users.

4 Understanding safety at work

It is important that you have a knowledge and understanding of the health and safety laws and regulations that affect how you carry out your work. It is equally important that you follow these laws and regulations. This chapter tells you about the laws and regulations that apply to working in care and how you should put them into practice. It builds on what you have learnt about the principles of care, your workplace policies and procedures and your role as a worker.

Successful completion of the activities in this chapter will enable you to demonstrate your understanding of the Induction Standard *Maintain safety at work*. It will also give you an opportunity to develop evidence for key skills unit Communication at level 1.

What is covered in this chapter?

This chapter contributes to the knowledge and understanding you need for the following NVQ Care units:

CU1 : Promote, monitor and maintain health, safety and security in the workplace
CU3 : Monitor and maintain the cleanliness of environments
NC12 : Help clients to eat and drink
NC13 : Prepare food and drink for clients
Z7   : Contribute to the movement and handling of clients to maximise their physical comfort

4.1 HEALTH AND SAFETY

Maintaining a healthy and safe workplace

The Health and Safety at Work Act 1974 is the most important workplace health and safety law. Its purpose is to protect the health and safety of everyone in the workplace. It describes the rights and responsibilities of employers and workers in making sure that the workplace is safe and healthy.

Workplace risk assessments are checks to find out how safe the workplace is. One of your employer's main responsibilities under the Health and Safety at Work Act is to carry out risk assessments and to make the workplace as safe as possible. Risk assessments lead to safety policies being written that describe, for example:

- training you need so that you can do your job safely
- safe moving and handling techniques you should use
- when and how you should wear protective clothing
- how to help control the spread of infection
- how to use equipment safely.

It is your responsibility to follow your employer's safety policies in your day-to-day work. By doing so, you will be protecting the health and safety of yourself, your colleagues and your service users.

Your responsibilities under the Health and Safety at Work Act are:

- to take care of everyone who may be affected by your work by:
  - only doing work you are trained to do
  - storing equipment properly
  - not fooling around or taking chances or short cuts

- to report health and safety hazards to your supervisor without delay, including:
  - faulty equipment and safety signs that have been tampered with
  - blocked exits and escape routes (stairwells, fire doors)
  - infectious diseases, injuries and accidents
- to help your employer carry out their health and safety responsibilities by:
  - following workplace health and safety procedures
  - not tampering with anything provided for your health and safety
  - knowing what to do in an emergency such as a fire
  - using protective clothing and equipment correctly.

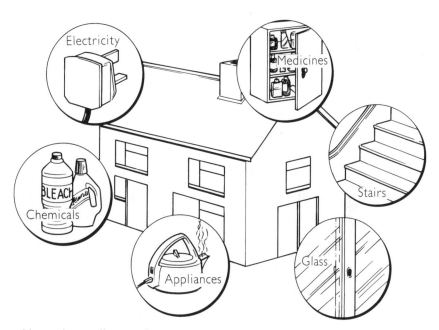

Potential hazards are all around us

What do you think?

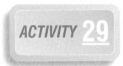

Carry out a survey of your workplace. Identify what you think may be health and safety hazards and say how you think you can help make the workplace more safe.

Health and safety hazards at work	How I could make the workplace more safe

Discuss your thoughts with your supervisor.

Protecting yourself from violence

Violence against care workers includes verbal abuse, harassment, threatening behaviour and assault. It ranges from minor incidents through to murder.

In order to protect yourself from violence, you need to know:

- which service users can become violent
- the sorts of situations that can lead to violence
- how to reduce the dangers.

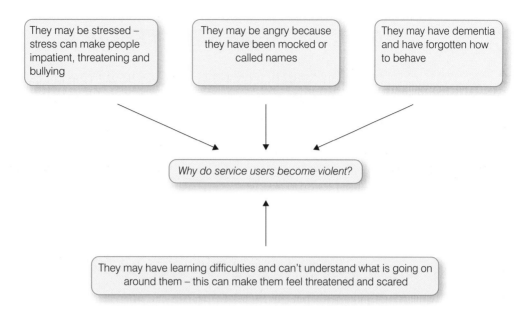

They may be stressed – stress can make people impatient, threatening and bullying

They may be angry because they have been mocked or called names

They may have dementia and have forgotten how to behave

Why do service users become violent?

They may have learning difficulties and can't understand what is going on around them – this can make them feel threatened and scared

Situations that might be a risk for you include those where:

- you are working alone, e.g. in the home of a confused service user
- you are working in a care setting with a number of adults with severe learning difficulties or dementia
- violent behaviour is rare and you aren't expecting it.

You can help reduce the dangers by:

- following your workplace's procedures for preventing and dealing with violence
- knowing what triggers violence and the signs that service users are becoming violent, e.g. shouting, fear, anxiety, confusion, anger, alcohol abuse
- regularly re-assessing the risk of violence – ask yourself questions about your behaviour and the effect it has on service users
- attending training on safe working methods and making sure that you use them at all times
- reporting any violent incidents promptly to your supervisor and recording them accurately in an incident book.

DEVELOP GOOD WORK PRACTICE (i) 4.2.2

ACTIVITY 30

Read your workplace's procedure on how to protect yourself from violence. Make brief notes on what it tells you.

_____

_____

_____

_____

_____

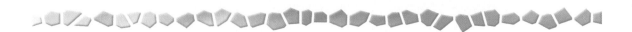

Emergencies with mains services

Mains services are gas, electricity and water supplies. Dangerous situations and emergencies can occur if there is a problem with mains services.

Gas leaks

Because gas is flammable, leaks can lead to fires and explosions. They can also cause breathing problems, unconsciousness and death (asphyxiation). Your workplace will have a procedure for dealing with gas leaks but as a general rule:

- open windows and doors to let the gas escape
- turn off fires and cookers and don't light matches or cigarette lighters
- turn the gas off at the mains supply (usually near the gas meter)
- telephone the emergency number of the gas company from an outside phone (in case using the workplace phone would cause an explosion)

- give first aid to anybody who is having difficulty breathing or dial 999 if there is a health emergency.

Electricity emergencies

Power surges, exposed wires, frayed cables, faulty switches and electrical appliances are also fire risks. Electricity can cause injuries such as shock, burns and asphyxiation. Again, your workplace will have a procedure for responding to electrical emergencies but as a general rule:

- turn the electricity supply off at the mains (usually near the fuse box)
- never touch a person or object that is connected to the electrical supply
- if somebody has had an electric shock, dial 999 or get help from a GP.

Your first aid training will show you how to help people who have difficulty breathing or who have had an electric shock.

Water leaks

Water leaks can rot floorboards and floor coverings, making them hazardous. When water comes into contact with electricity there is a risk of fire and electrical injuries. Your workplace will have a procedure to follow in the event of an water leak, but as a general rule:

- put a bucket, bowl or towel under the leak
- turn the water supply off at the stopcock (usually near a sink)
- if water is leaking from the main water tank, leave bath taps turned on to empty the tank
- call the emergency number of the water company
- mop up as best you can.

Let your supervisor know what you have done. He or she will take over responsibility for dealing with the situation.

DEVELOP GOOD WORK PRACTICE 4.2.3

ACTIVITY 31

Find out where your workplace gas, electricity and water mains switches and stopcocks are and make a note of their location.

- gas mains switch: _____
- electricity mains switch: _____
- water stopcock: _____

Ask someone to show you how to turn them off.

Find out and write down the names and emergency phone numbers of the companies that supply your workplace with gas, electricity and water.

- gas supplier and emergency number: _____
- electricity supplier and emergency number: _____
- water supplier and emergency number: _____

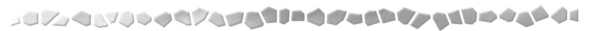

Working safely with hazardous substances

The Control of Substances Hazardous to Health (COSHH) Regulations 1994 set out to protect people when they are working with hazardous or harmful substances.

Hazardous substances you might come into contact with and their effect on health

Hazardous substances	Examples	Health effects
Cleaning materials	Bleach, disinfectant	Skin problems, e.g. burns, dermatitis Breathing problems, e.g. asthma
Body fluids and waste	Urine, faeces, blood, vomit	Infections
Clinical waste	Used dressings	Infections
Sharps	Needles, syringes	Wounds and infections
Soiled linen	Sheets, clothing	Infections

Your workplace obeys the COSHH Regulations by having a COSHH file. You have a responsibility to read the file and work to the procedures it gives you. In this way you will be helping to protect everyone's health and safety.

The COSHH file tells you:

- what protective clothing you must wear when you work with hazardous substances, e.g. gloves and aprons
- how to store hazardous substances, e.g. in correctly labelled containers with safety lids
- how to dispose of hazardous substances. For example:
  - body fluids and waste must be flushed down the sluice drain
  - clinical waste must be put in a labelled yellow bag and sent for incineration
  - sharps must be put in a yellow sharps box and sent for incineration
  - soiled linen must be put in red bags and sent to the laundry
  - unused medication should be returned to the pharmacist.

CHECK YOUR UNDERSTANDING

 4.2.4

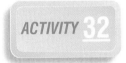

Complete the table to show your understanding of how to work with hazardous substances. You might need to read the COSHH file to help with your entries.

Check with your supervisor that your understanding is correct.

Hazardous substances I work with	Precautions I should take when using these substances	Precautions I should take when storing these substances	Precautions I should take when disposing of these substances

Security at work

Locking and chaining doors, locking windows, being careful about who we give our personal details to and installing burglar alarms are some of the safety measures we can take to maintain our security. Feeling secure means feeling safe and feeling safe is important for good health and well-being.

Service users also need to feel safe and they have a right to be secure. For this reason, your workplace will have various safety measures and procedures in place and it is your responsibility to:

- politely check the identity of visitors to your workplace. Ask to see some proof of identity such as an ID badge. Confirm with your supervisor that they have a right to visit before you let them in

- check that people at your workplace want to see any visitors who call. Not all visitors are welcome

- make sure that visitors are given a name badge and that they complete the visitors book on arrival and when they leave

- know who should and shouldn't be in the workplace and raise the alarm if you discover an intruder.

Other security measures include burglar alarms and panic buttons. Make sure you know how they work and that you use them properly. Don't take chances.

DEVELOP GOOD WORK PRACTICE 4.2.5

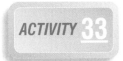

Talk to your supervisor about the safety measures at your workplace. List them below.

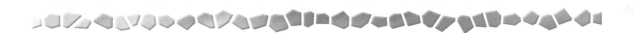

4.2 MOVING AND HANDLING

Know your back!

About one in three injuries at work are caused by moving and handling, e.g. carrying, pushing, lifting or lowering a load. A load can be a cup of tea; it can also be a service user. About half of these moving and handling injuries affect the back. They can cause pain, slipped discs, even paralysis. Care workers are more likely to be involved in moving and handling than most other workers, so you can see how risky your job is!

In order to avoid moving and handling back injuries, you should understand how your back works and how it can be injured.

The backbone or spine is made up of 33 small bones called <u>vertebrae.</u> The way they are joined together gives us an S-shaped posture. This 'S' shape gives our backs 'spring' and strength and helps us to keep our balance. If moving and handling activities cause the spine to change its shape, e.g. by twisting down at the waist to pick something up, it becomes weak and easily injured.

The spine protects the <u>spinal cord</u> (a bundle of nerves) that 'runs' through the vertebrae from the bottom of the spine to the brain. The spinal cord carries 'messages' from the muscles to the brain and from the brain to the muscles. Damage to the spine can damage the spinal cord, sometimes resulting in paralysis.

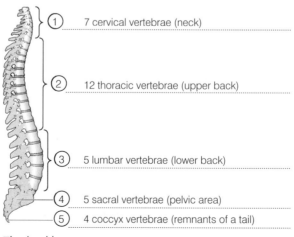

1. 7 cervical vertebrae (neck)

2. 12 thoracic vertebrae (upper back)

3. 5 lumbar vertebrae (lower back)

4. 5 sacral vertebrae (pelvic area)

5. 4 coccyx vertebrae (remnants of a tail)

The backbone

Between the vertebrae are intervertebral discs. These are cushion-like structures that act as shock absorbers and enable the vertebrae to move. If moving and handling activities put too much pressure on intervertebral discs, e.g. by bending backwards to put something up on a shelf, they can tear (prolapsed or 'slipped' disc). Slipped discs are extremely painful.

Spinal ligaments are springy structures that link the vertebrae together. If a manual handling activity causes ligaments to be overstretched, e.g. through supporting a service user for a longish period of time, or to be stretched at high speed, e.g. moving jerkily to catch someone before they fall, ligaments can sprain and become swollen and painful.

The muscles of the spine are the muscles of the back, chest and pelvis (the hip area of the skeleton) that are attached to the vertebrae. Together, these muscles strengthen the spine and allow it to move. Strong, well-toned spinal muscles are necessary for moving and handling activities. Weak muscles are easily torn, becoming swollen and painful.

CHECK YOUR UNDERSTANDING 4.1.1

ACTIVITY 34

Produce an information sheet for your colleagues that:

1 lists the different parts of the spine
2 describes how moving and handling activities can cause back injuries.

Moving and handling and the law

The purpose of moving and handling law is to prevent moving and handling injuries. There are a number of laws and regulations which tell us how to prevent moving and handling injuries at work.

Manual Handling Operations Regulations (MHOR) 1992. These describe procedures to follow to reduce moving and handling injuries

Management of Health and Safety at Work Regulations (MHSWR) 1992. These look at the risks involved with moving and handling and how they should be dealt with

Moving and Handling Laws and Regulations

Lifting Operations and Lifting Equipment Regulations (LOLER) 1999 and Provisions and Use of Work Equipment Regulations (PUWER) 1999. These are concerned with workplace moving and handling equipment

Reporting of Injuries, Diseases and Dangerous Occurrences Regulations (RIDDOR) 1995. These describe what to do in the event of a workplace accident or injury

DEVELOP GOOD WORK PRACTICE

4.1.2

ACTIVITY 35

Read your workplace policy on moving and handling and make a list of the moving and handling regulations that influence the way you do your job.

_____

_____

_____

_____

_____

_____

_____

_____

_____

_____

Moving and handling risk assessments

A moving and handling risk assessment is a check to see:

- how loads are moved and handled
- whether the moving and handling can be changed to make it more safe.

All moving and handling activities in your workplace will have been 'risk-assessed'. It is your responsibility to carry out moving and handling activities as the risk assessment tells you.

There are five stages to a risk assessment.

1 First of all, the person doing the risk assessment would ask 'Is this moving and handling activity risky in any way?' The Health and Safety Executive (HSE) has published a set of guidelines that can be used to help decide whether an activity is risky or not.

2 If they think that the activity is risky, they would then ask 'Who might be harmed and how?'

3 Next they would decide either to get rid of the risky activity or to change it to one that is less harmful. This is called 'controlling the risks'.

4 A record is then written that lets people know that the activity has been assessed for risks and how it must be carried out so that it is as risk-free as possible.

5 The risk assessor will then set a date to check that the new way of doing the activity is more safe or whether it needs further changes.

Risk assessments are common-sense procedures but they are very important if moving and handling injuries are to be prevented.

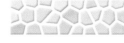

DEVELOP GOOD WORK PRACTICE

 4.1.3

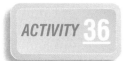

Read the risk assessments for two of the moving and handling activities that you are required to carry out. Make a note of the procedures they tell you to follow and explain why it is important that you follow these procedures.

Moving and handling activity	How I should carry out this activity	Why I should carry this activity out in this way

SAFER moving and handling techniques

There are five steps to **SAFER** moving and handling. However, before you are allowed to move and handle loads – which, don't forget, include service users – you will need to have attended a practical moving and handling training session (see Activity 37).

The 5 steps to **SAFER** moving and handling are:

1 **S**top and think. Should you be carrying out this moving and handling activity? Can you avoid it at all?

2 **A**ssess the situation. If you can't avoid the activity, you must follow the procedure given in the risk assessment. But, because situations are never quite as they should be, think about your situation before you start the activity. Do you need to get help, to use any equipment or to improve the space you are working in?

3 **F**ormulate an action plan. Once you have assessed your situation you can plan how you are going to carry out the activity.

4 **E**xecute or carry out your plan. When carrying out a moving and handling activity, move the following parts of your body in a smooth and co-ordinated way:

   Your feet – Keep your feet as close to your load as possible, slightly apart and with one just in front of the other

   Your legs – Bend your knees and hips slightly

   Your back – Stand close to your load and maintain an S-shaped posture; don't twist to lift from the side or stoop to lift from in front; when pushing, lean slightly into your load, and when pulling, lean slightly away

   Your arms and hands – Use your arms to keep your load close to your body; keep your elbows bent and tucked in to your side; and use your hands, not your fingers, to grasp your load

   Your head – Keep your chin raised and look straight ahead

   Working with a colleague and encouraging service users to move more independently lightens your load

5 **R**eview the way you carried out the activity. Did things go to plan? If not, why not? How can you change the moving and handling activity to reduce the effort and discomfort for all concerned?

By following these five steps to SAFER moving and handling you can ensure your own personal health and safety as well as that of your colleagues and service users.

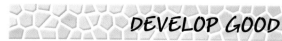 **DEVELOP GOOD WORK PRACTICE** 4.1.4, 4.1.5

ACTIVITY 37

Complete the following details:

The Moving and Handling training I attended took place on _____

My Moving and Handling Certificate can be found _____

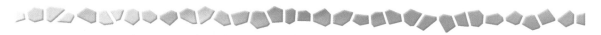

4.3 FIRE SAFETY

Fires kill hundreds of people every year even though most of them can be prevented.

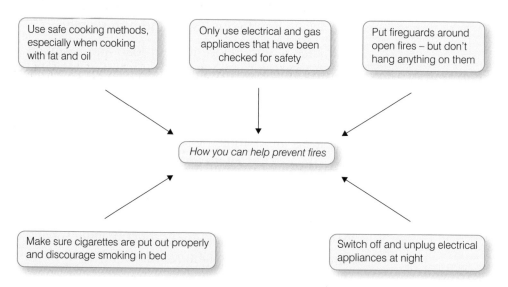

Use safe cooking methods, especially when cooking with fat and oil

Only use electrical and gas appliances that have been checked for safety

Put fireguards around open fires – but don't hang anything on them

How you can help prevent fires

Make sure cigarettes are put out properly and discourage smoking in bed

Switch off and unplug electrical appliances at night

Ways to prevent fires from spreading include:

- using fire-proof furnishings and bedding
- keeping windows and doors closed – fire doors must ALWAYS be kept closed
- using smoke alarms. These alert you to a fire before it spreads. Some smoke alarms have flashing lights or vibrating pads and so are valuable if people have difficulty seeing or hearing.

Your workplace fire safety procedures are based on the Fire Precautions (Workplace) Regulations 1997. All workplaces are different because they are built differently and have different types of people working and living in them. For this reason all workplaces have different fire safety procedures.

It is very important that you know your workplace's procedures for fire safety and that you attend fire safety training at least once a year. However, a general checklist is as follows.

- If you discover a fire, raise the alarm. Use the fire alarm or shout for help. If you are asked to call in the emergency services, dial 999, ask for the fire service and describe clearly where the fire is. Don't hang up until the address has been repeated back to you

- Close windows and doors to prevent fire and smoke spreading

- If service users can move, help them to a part of the building that is safe or to the assembly point outside. Always use the fire exits and fire escape route

- If service users can't move, it might be more sensible for them to remain where they are and be rescued by the fire service

- Close doors as you pass through them, don't stop for any reason and don't use the lifts

- Be calm, don't panic and don't rush

- Check that everyone is accounted for. The fire service will need to know where everyone is

- Don't return to the building until the fire service gives the OK.

If it is safe to do so, you might be able to put a fire out yourself. Your workplace may have fire blankets. These are used for smothering flames on solids, liquids, chip pans and people. Read the instructions before you attempt to use them.

Your workplace may also be fitted out with fire extinguishers. As all extinguishers will eventually be red you must read the instructions to find out how to use them and what types of fire they are for.

Contents	Types of fire it can be used for
Water	Wood, cloth and paper fires but not electrical, fat or oil fires (**not** chip pan fires)
Carbon dioxide	Electrical fires and burning liquids
Dry powder	Burning liquids and solids and electrical fires
Foam	Burning liquids and petrol fires
Halon	Electrical fires, burning liquids and small solid fires
AFFF	General fires and burning liquids

It is very helpful for service users to know fire safety procedures. You can teach them about fire safety by:

- explaining the meaning of different alarms and fire safety signs, e.g. fire alarms, fire exits, fire escape routes. If you work with people who have a sight or hearing impairment, your workplace will have adapted signs and alarms, e.g. signs in braille, flashing lights, vibrating buttons. Make sure everyone knows what these mean
- showing videos and having discussions about what to do in case of fire
- having regular fire drills to make sure that everyone recognises the fire alarm, knows how to walk away from a fire without panicking and knows how to help others who are confused or have mobility problems.

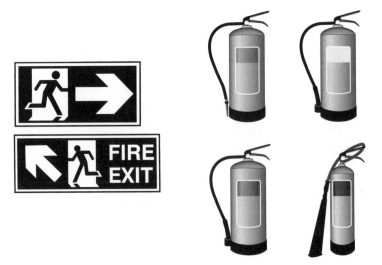

Fire safety equipment

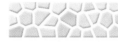

DEVELOP GOOD WORK PRACTICE

 4.3.1

ACTIVITY 38

1 Complete the following details:

The Fire Safety Training I attended took place on _____

My Fire Safety Training Certificate can be found _____

2 Make brief notes on the fire safety procedures for your workplace

_____

_____

_____

_____

_____

_____

_____

3 List the ways that your workplace ensures that service users are familiar with fire safety procedures.

_____

_____

_____

_____

_____

_____

_____

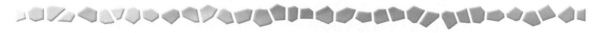

4.4 EMERGENCY FIRST AID

Your workplace's procedures for dealing with first aid emergencies are based on the Health and Safety (First Aid) Regulations 1981. It is very important that you know and follow these procedures and that you attend first aid training and refresher courses on a regular basis.

Your role in emergency first aid situations

First aid is a skill that requires training and practice. The aims of first aid are to:

- **p**reserve a casualty's life
- **p**revent further harm
- **p**romote (help) their recovery.

If you haven't yet attended first aid training, you shouldn't attempt to give anything more than the basic first aid described below. If you have been on a first aid course in a previous job or at school and your first aid certificate is up to date, you may be competent (skilled) in giving artificial ventilation and cardiopulmonary resuscitation (CPR). However, only give first aid that you know you can do safely and with confidence.

Basic first aid for emergencies – DR ABC

D is for DANGER

Before giving help of any kind, check the situation for danger to yourself. Don't attempt to help if helping would put you in danger. Don't delay in sending for qualified help.

R is for RESPONSE

Try to get a response from the casualty. Talk to them and gently shake their shoulders. If they are conscious and respond to you in a normal way, reassure them that help is on its way. Move them to a safer place if there is a risk of further injury. If they don't respond, continue to talk to them and to gently shake their shoulders.

A is for AIRWAY

If the casualty is unconscious or responds to you with difficulty, your priority is to check that their airway – mouth and throat – is not blocked. A blocked airway leads to choking and suffocation. If you can, remove the cause of the blockage, taking care not to push it further down the throat. Open the airway by tilting the casualty's head backwards and lifting their chin. Check that qualified help is on its way.

B is for BREATHING

Check that the casualty is breathing. You can do this by putting your cheek close to their mouth and looking down over their chest, watching for breathing movements. If they are breathing, put them into the recovery position. This keeps the airway open. You will practise putting someone into the recovery position in your first aid course.

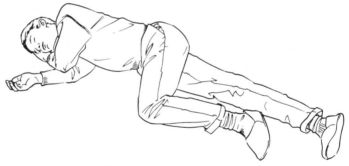

The recovery position ensures that the casualty's airway is open

If the casualty is not breathing, check that qualified help is on the way. **If you are competent**, give artificial ventilation. You will learn how to give artificial ventilation in your first aid course.

C is for CIRCULATION

Check whether the casualty's heart is beating. You can do this by feeling for their pulse. You will practise checking for a pulse in your first aid course.

If the casualty doesn't have a pulse or a heartbeat (cardiac arrest), check that help is on the way. **If you are competent** give cardiopulmonary resuscitation (CPR). You will learn how to give CPR in your first aid course.

It is very important that you only give first aid that you know you can do safely. By doing something you're not competent and confident to do you can make things worse for the casualty. If you're not sure what to do, send for someone who is competent and help them in whatever way they ask.

The following first aid techniques are basic and common sense. However, once you have given help you should still summon support from a competent person.

Minor wounds and bleeding	Wash your hands. Tie a clean dressing (from the first aid box if possible) firmly over the casualty's wound. If the bleeding continues, put another dressing on top of the first one and get help
Suspected broken bones (fractures)	Don't move the casualty unless they are in a dangerous position. Get help
Burns and scalds	Cool with cold water. Get help
Eye injuries	Wash your hands. Wash the casualty's eye with clean, cool water. Don't attempt to remove anything from the eye

You will learn how to deal with severe bleeding, more complicated wounds, broken bones and serious burns and scalds in your first aid course

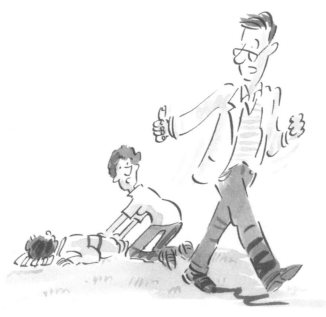

If you are unable to give first aid safely, ask someone to fetch help

Under the Reporting of Injuries, Diseases and Dangerous Occurrences Regulations (RIDDOR) 1995, accidents and injuries that happen at work, and the treatment that is given, must be recorded in the Accident Book. This sort of information is needed to help identify health and safety risks so that they can be reduced or eliminated (got rid of).

DEVELOP GOOD WORK PRACTICE 4.4.1, 4.4.2

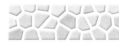
ACTIVITY 39

Complete the following details:

The First Aid Training I attended took place on _____

First aid I am qualified to give now _____

First aid I am not yet qualified to give _____

My First Aid Certificate can be found _____

I need to renew my First Aid Certificate on _____

My workplace's Accident Book can be found _____

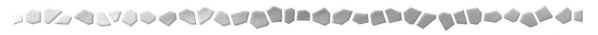

Primary health care services

Primary health care services are provided by GPs, nurses, dentists, opticians and pharmacists. These are the people we go to first in the event of an accident or ill health.

GPs diagnose and treat illnesses, prescribe medicines, give advice and refer patients to specialist consultants if necessary. They also carry out minor surgery. If a service user becomes ill, you should telephone their GP surgery but if there is a first aid emergency you should dial 999 for an ambulance. When you dial 999 it is important that you are able to answer clearly and calmly questions about:

- the casualty, such as their name and age
- the location of the emergency – the address and telephone number

- the cause of the emergency
- what first aid has already been given.

If you are unsure about the seriousness of an illness or injury, there may be an NHS Drop In Centre nearby where you can take the casualty for advice or treatment. You could also telephone NHS Direct and talk your concerns through with an expert.

Dentists work in hospitals and in the community. They do check-ups, fillings, extractions, X-rays and fit bridges and dentures. Opticians examine eyes, prescribe treatment and fit glasses and contact lenses. Pharmacists or chemists give advice, supply medicines for minor illnesses and prescriptions and give instructions for the use of medicines. These professionals are also able to respond to emergencies and you must be able to find the contact details of your service users' dentists, opticians and chemists.

DEVELOP GOOD WORK PRACTICE 4.4.3

ACTIVITY 40

1 Note down where you can find contact details of your service users' GPs, dentists, opticians and chemists

_____

_____

_____

2 Make a note of the address of your nearest NHS Drop In Centre and the telephone number for NHS Direct.

_____

_____

_____

_____

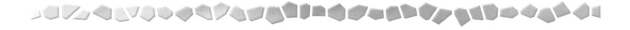

4.5 SAFE FOOD HANDLING

Your workplace's procedures for safe food handling are based on the Food Safety Act 1990 and the Food Safety (General Food Hygiene) Regulations 1995. It is very important that you know and use food safety procedures and that you attend food hygiene training sessions.

Food that is handled unsafely can become contaminated (spoiled) by bacteria, viruses and fungi. If we eat food that has been contaminated, we are likely to get food poisoning.

The symptoms of food poisoning are feeling sick (nausea), stomach pains, diarrhoea and vomiting. Frail and elderly service users are most at risk of food poisoning. It is therefore your responsibility to know what causes food poisoning and how it can be prevented. By doing so you can make sure that food is handled safely and so protect service users' health and safety.

What causes food poisoning?

Name of bacteria	Where the bacteria are found
Staphylococcus aureus (S. aureus)	On our skin, in our nose, throat, mouth, ears, hair, nails, and in wounds such as cuts and boils. S. aureus is relatively harmless until it is transferred to food, when it produces poisons (toxins)
Escherichia coli (E. coli)	Our intestines and our faeces. E. coli is also harmless until it is transferred to food
Salmonella and Clostridium perfringens	Raw meat, poultry, eggs, shellfish and sometimes human faeces

As well as growing in raw food and being carried by humans, food poisoning bacteria are found in:

- pets and pests – for example, dogs, cats, birds, insects, mice and rats (rodents) carry bacteria on their bodies and in their urine and faeces
- rotting rubbish and waste food
- our clothes and jewellery.

Preventing food poisoning

Food poisoning can be avoided by preventing the spread of bacteria to food.

Preventing the spread of bacteria to food through good personal hygiene

If you are involved in the handling of food:

- Wash your hands with soap and water before handling food
- Wash your hands with soap and water after using the toilet and helping service users use the toilet, handling raw food and rubbish, coughing, sneezing, using a handkerchief and touching your face or hair
- Wear the protective clothing you are given
- Keep your nails short and clean and don't wear nail varnish or jewellery
- Keep your hair clean and tied back or covered
- Keep wounds covered with coloured waterproof dressings and check that you are allowed to handle food when wearing a dressing
- Don't smoke in a food area – it is against the law!

If you or anyone you live with is unwell, you must tell your supervisor. It may be that you will not be allowed to work with food for the time being.

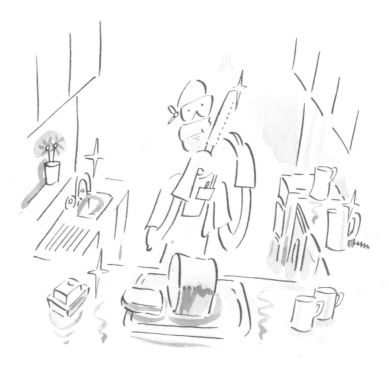

Hygiene is extremely important when preparing food

Preventing the spread of bacteria to food by other food and equipment

- Store raw and cooked foods in different fridges
- If there is only one fridge, store raw foods on lower shelves than cooked foods
- Use different work surfaces for preparing raw and cooked foods
- Use different equipment, e.g. knives, chopping boards and wiping cloths, for raw and cooked foods, and store them separately
- Keep work surfaces, equipment and wiping cloths thoroughly clean, especially after using them for raw meat and poultry
- Keep food covered
- Don't use food that is past its 'use by' date

Preventing the spread of bacteria to food by pets and pests

- Check for pets and pests in the food storage, kitchen and eating areas and call the Environmental Health Department for advice if you see signs of an infestation, e.g. droppings
- Throw out any food that might have been spoiled by pets or pests
- Keep up a high standard of cleanliness – sweep floors, wipe up spills, wash and store equipment properly
- Keep doors and windows closed, use fly screens
- Keep food and waste covered and empty waste bins regularly

You can also help prevent the spread of bacteria by storing and cooking food at the right temperatures:

- **70°C and above** – Most bacteria are killed at this heat so cook foods thoroughly
- **5°C to 63°C** – the Temperature Danger Zone! Most bacteria thrive in the Temperature Danger Zone so store food below 5°C or above 63°C
- **–22°C to 5°C** – Most bacteria can't grow at these low temperatures so check that fridges and freezers stay within these limits.

The Reporting of Injuries, Diseases and Dangerous Occurrences (RIDDOR) Regulations state that your employer must notify the local Environmental Health Department of any cases of food poisoning in your workplace. Your workplace procedure will outline any responsibilities you have in completing reports and records.

CHECK YOUR UNDERSTANDING

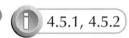 4.5.1, 4.5.2

ACTIVITY 41

1 List the three main causes of food poisoning

_____

_____

_____

_____

2 Talk to the team at your workplace who are responsible for food storage, preparation and handling. Jot down the procedures they follow to protect service users and colleagues from food poisoning.

_____

_____

_____

_____

_____

_____

3 Complete the following details:

The Food Hygiene Training I attended took place on _____

My Food Hygiene Certificate can be found _____

4.6 INFECTION CONTROL

Your service users may be elderly, have disabilities, be experiencing ill health or live in unhealthy surroundings. Because of this, they are at risk of catching infectious diseases. Your workplace will have procedures for making sure that the spread of infection is controlled. It is your responsibility to know and follow these infection control procedures so that the health and safety of service users is protected.

Some infectious diseases and their causes

Infectious diseases	Causes of the diseases
Sore throats, boils, pneumonia, tuberculosis (TB), tetanus, impetigo, gastroenteritis, methicillin-resistant _Staphylococcus aureus_ (MRSA)	Bacteria
Influenza (flu), colds, mumps, herpes (e.g. cold sores), hepatitis B	Viruses
Thrush (_Candida_), ringworm	Fungi

Infestations are caused by animals such as head lice, pubic lice and mites. Mites that burrow into the skin to lay their eggs cause scabies, sometimes known as 'the itch'.

The Reporting of Injuries, Diseases and Dangerous Occurrences (RIDDOR) Regulations state that your employer must notify the local Environmental Health Department if certain infectious diseases occur in the workplace. Your workplace's infection control procedure will outline your responsibilities in completing reports and records.

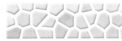 *DEVELOP GOOD WORK PRACTICE* 4.6.3

ACTIVITY 42

Find out from your supervisor and list the infectious diseases:

1 that have been experienced by service users and colleagues in your workplace

_____

_____

_____

_____

_____

_____

2 that need to be reported to the Environmental Health Department.

_____

_____

_____

_____

_____

_____

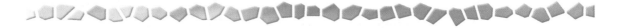

How are infectious diseases caught?

Ways that diseases are caught	Examples of diseases
Direct contact (being touched by an infected person) Indirect contact (touching things such as handkerchiefs and towels that an infected person has used) Diseases spread by direct and indirect skin contact are known as <u>contagious diseases</u>	Scabies, ringworm, impetigo, herpes
Inhaling (breathing in) the droplets sprayed out when an infected person coughs or sneezes	Colds, influenza (flu), measles
Eating food and drink that has been contaminated by an infected person or animal	Gastroenteritis
Using health-care instruments such as needles after they have been used on an infected person	AIDS, hepatitis B

CHECK YOUR UNDERSTANDING

 4.6.2

ACTIVITY 43

Make notes on how two or three of the infectious diseases you listed for Activity 42 are caught.

_____

_____

_____

_____

_____

_____

Preventing the spread of infection

Infection can be prevented from spreading (controlled) in a number of ways. The most important way is to help your service users stay healthy by making sure that they eat well, are immunised against infectious diseases such as flu and take their medication as prescribed.

You can also help prevent the spread of infection by following workplace procedures and manufacturer's instructions, especially when you are:

- working with service users who have particular types of infectious disease
- cleaning, disinfecting and sterilising equipment
- cleaning up spillages and dealing with waste.

Effective hand washing

Another very important method of preventing the spread of infection is to:

- wash your hands with soap and water before
  - handling food
  - giving medication
  - giving first aid and handling wounds
- wash your hands with soap and water after
  - using the toilet and helping others to use the toilet
  - coughing, sneezing, using a handkerchief, touching faces, hair, dentures
  - giving first aid and handling wounds
  - making beds
  - handling raw food and rubbish
  - handling equipment, laundry and waste contaminated with body fluids.

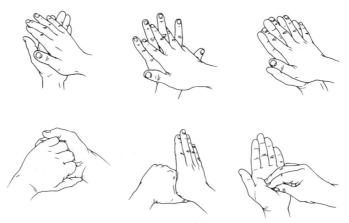

Correct handwashing technique

You need to learn and practise the correct technique for washing your hands:

1 Wet your hands with hot running water and rub some soap between your palms

2 Rub your right palm over the back of your left hand and then your left palm over the back of your right hand

3 Rub your palms together again but this time with your fingers interlocked

4 Rub the back of the fingers of your left hand with your right palm and then the back of the fingers of your right hand with your left palm

5 Rub around your left thumb with your right palm and then around your right thumb with your left palm

6 Rub your left fingertips round and round in your right palm then your right fingertips round and round in your left palm

7 Rub your left wrist with your right hand then your right wrist with your left hand

8 Rinse both hands thoroughly under running water and dry them carefully on clean paper towels.

You should wash your hands even if you have been wearing gloves.

DEVELOP GOOD WORK PRACTICE 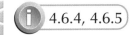 4.6.4, 4.6.5

ACTIVITY 44

1 Practise washing your hands as described above and ask your supervisor to observe you to make sure that you are washing them effectively.

_____ [name of worker] has demonstrated to me that s/he knows how to wash his/her hands effectively.

Signed: _____ Date: _____

[name of supervisor]

2 Make a list of other procedures you use that help prevent the spread of infectious diseases.

_____

_____

_____

_____

_____

_____

_____

_____

Wearing protective clothing

The Personal Protective Equipment (PPE) Regulations 1992 state that your employer must provide you with protective clothing. Protective clothing is important because it prevents cross-infection, i.e. it prevents you from being infected by your service users and prevents them from being infected by you.

You must wear protective clothing every time you come into contact with body fluids and waste, e.g. blood, saliva, mucus (from the nose and lungs), urine, faeces and vomit. Aprons or overalls prevent infection from wastes and body fluids spreading on to your clothes and then spreading on to the next person you work with. You should wear a clean apron or overall for every service user you work with. Plastic aprons are a good idea because they are disposable.

If you have to work with body fluids and waste and with wounds, pressure sores, rashes, dressings and soiled linen, you must wear gloves. Gloves protect your hands from infection and prevent infection spreading from you to the next person you work with. Gloves should be thrown away after being used and you should wash your hands after wearing them.

CHECK YOUR UNDERSTANDING

4.6.6

ACTIVITY 45

Make notes to describe the protective clothing you are required to wear, when you would wear it and why.

_____

_____

_____

_____

_____

_____

_____

_____

DEVELOP GOOD WORK PRACTICE

4.6.1

ACTIVITY 46

Carry out a survey of two or three different areas in your workplace, e.g. the dining area, a bathroom, a bedroom. Make a list of the infection risks that you think are present in each area.

_____

_____

_____

_____

_____

_____

_____

_____

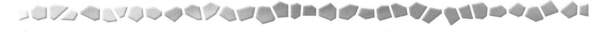

5 Understanding the effects of the care service setting on providing services

If you have experience of working in different types of employment, you will know that different workplaces and job roles affect workers in different ways. A workplace that delivers care also has an effect on the users of its services. This chapter aims to develop your understanding about how workplaces that deliver care – care service settings – affect both care workers and service users.

Successful completion of the activities in this chapter will enable you to demonstrate your understanding of the Induction Standard *Understand the effects of the service setting on providing services*. It will also give you an opportunity to develop evidence for key skills unit Communication at level 1.

What is covered in this chapter?

This chapter builds on what you have learnt in the previous four chapters and contributes to the knowledge and understanding you need for the following NVQ Care units:

CU10 : Contribute to the effectiveness of work teams

W3 : Support individuals experiencing a change in their care requirements and provision

Z8 : Support individuals when they are distressed

5.1 THE EFFECTS OF THE CARE SERVICE SETTING ON SERVICE USERS

We are all individuals, each with our own unique life history and experiences, preferred ways of doing things, hopes and expectations. Good care practice involves recognising and respecting service users' individuality in the way you work with and support them.

Whatever care service setting you are employed in, whether residential home, nursing home, day care centre or the service user's own home, you have a responsibility to develop and use good care practices – the care values – in your work.

> *CASE STUDY: Maggie*
>
> *Maggie has recently moved into residential care because, as a result of a stroke, she needs help to move around, to eat and drink and to care for her personal hygiene. The stroke also affected her sight and she has problems with remembering recent events. She has had to sell her house and many treasured possessions to help pay for her care.*

How do you think Maggie might feel about these changes in her circumstances?

As regards having to move into a residential care setting, she may be troubled about having to get on with people she doesn't know and may not like. She may be worried about the timing of meals and having to eat food she doesn't enjoy. She may be concerned that she won't be able to entertain her friends in private or go and visit her family when she wishes.

She may also be frustrated with her failure to be independent and her memory loss. She may be anxious because she can't see very well, ashamed that she needs help with private and personal matters and depressed that she is losing her dignity. She may be angry because she had no choice about having to sell things that mean a lot to her.

As Maggie's case study shows, changes in circumstances that result in people needing care can be very distressing for them. Being cared for can mean having to change the way they live their lives. Like Maggie, your service users may no longer be able to do things in the way they would like. Their hopes and expectations may have faded away. The experiences that mean so much to them and that have made them the people they are today may seem to have lost any importance. In other words, they may feel that they have lost their identity and individuality.

It is very important that you reassure service users who are experiencing changes in their care needs that you value them as individuals:

- explain why they need care – use words and body language that they understand and that show your understanding for how they feel
- encourage them to ask questions and tell you how they feel, e.g. about the service setting and the way they are to be given care
- encourage them to tell you how their likes and dislikes, views and beliefs can be respected in the way they are cared for, e.g. food preferences and religious beliefs
- know where to get help if you are unable to help them cope with the changes they are going through, e.g. counsellors, telephone helplines
- introduce them to other people they will come into contact with
- show them around so that they become familiar with their new surroundings and know where things are
- let them choose how to arrange their surroundings, e.g. using and arranging their own furniture, choosing the colour scheme and decorations
- with their permission, accurately report their views and concerns to your supervisor so that they can be dealt with.

It is also important to let your supervisor know how service users are coping with the care setting and to be flexible in the way you care. For example, if service users are becoming:

- forgetful – could you reintroduce people to each other?
- confused – could you show them around the care setting again?
- hard of hearing – can you change the way you communicate with them?

What do you think? 5.1.1

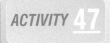 **CASE STUDY: Bill**

Bill is a new service user where you work. Note down three aspects of your workplace that might make him feel uncomfortable. For each aspect, briefly describe how you would help him feel more relaxed.

Aspects that might make Bill uncomfortable	How I could help him feel more relaxed
1	
2	
3	

5.2 THE EFFECTS OF THE CARE SERVICE SETTING ON THE WORKER

Supporting the care team

In Chapter 2, you read about the different teams of people who work in the caring services. You also identified the people in your team and looked at your and their roles and responsibilities as individual workers. This section looks at the responsibilities you and your team members have towards each other.

To work well as a team, members have to share a common goal. You might each have different tasks to perform but the common goal of the team is caring for and supporting service users.

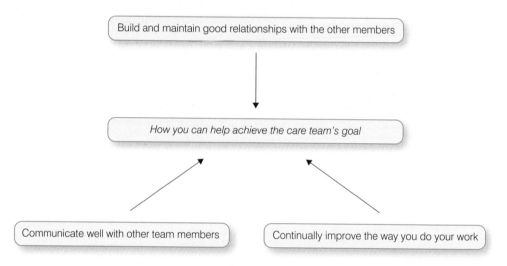

Relationships with team members are first and foremost working relationships. You don't have to be the best of friends with your colleagues but you do have a responsibility to offer each other assistance and support in a friendly and helpful way. Like service users, team members have a right to be respected and treated with consideration.

Team members also have a responsibility to be dependable, reliable, professional and trustworthy. Teams can't perform effectively if individual members arrive late for work, take time off for unacceptable reasons, don't work in a skilled way or neglect to do tasks they have promised to do. Behaviours like these, as well as personality clashes, name calling and bullying, lead to upset, resentment and breakdowns in relationships.

It is important for both the team and service users that work relationship problems are sorted out. There is usually a good reason why people behave 'out of line'. They may have problems at home, they may be stressed or they may simply be unaware that their behaviour is unacceptable. Talking calmly together as a team about the situation can be very useful but if this fails your supervisor will be able to give advice.

Communication is vital to good teamwork. Examples of the things team members have a responsibility to share with each other are:

- information that could be useful to the team or individual members
- ideas about how the team could improve the way it works
- ideas about how team members could improve the way they work
- any problems they are having doing their work
- information about what they will be doing, where and when.

Good communication means sharing ideas and information clearly and helpfully. Differences in opinion should be respected so that there is no conflict and no-one takes offence. Pre-arranged team meetings are the

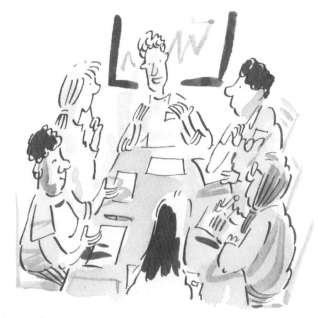

Sharing thoughts and experiences is beneficial to the team

best time to exchange information and ideas, not when people are busy or seem to have more important things on their minds.

Good communication means listening to what team members have to say, including any feedback they give you about how you are doing your job. Feedback should always be helpful and, by acting on it, you will help improve the way the team works together.

Finally, good communication requires that you know and understand your colleagues, their personalities and their backgrounds. Use appropriate words and body language, e.g. not slang, jargon (technical words) or humour they won't understand, or touch if it makes them uncomfortable. Make every effort to understand what they say to you.

What do you think?

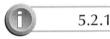 5.2.1

ACTIVITY 48

Think of a situation in which your team works well together.

1 List the factors that you think enable the team to work well together

_____

_____

_____

_____

_____

2 Describe what you think would happen if team members didn't work well together

_____

_____

_____

_____

_____

Working alone

Even though you are part of a care team, team work doesn't always mean being with your colleagues. There may be times when you will be on your own, e.g. in a service user's home or travelling between visits. Lone working can be quite difficult at first. It is your responsibility to be aware of possible problems and to know how to reduce or avoid them.

Working without your colleagues close by can knock your self-confidence. Because they are not there to support you, you might start to feel isolated and to wonder whether you are doing a task correctly. The solution to this problem is to make sure you are well trained and practised in giving care before you go out on your own. Also, check that you know who you should contact if you get into difficulty.

If you have appointments to keep with service users in their own homes, you need to develop good time management skills. Not sticking to your schedule can be hard when service users want to talk. However, staying longer than planned means you will be late for the next appointment. If you develop good working relationships with service users, they will understand that you have to work to a timetable.

Working in service users' own homes can put your health and safety at risk. For example, there is the risk of catching infections from towels, bed linen, pets and pests. You could be injured when using electrical equipment. Service users can be demanding and difficult, perhaps even abusive. Before you go out on your own, make sure you know your workplace's procedures for protecting yourself from risks and that you are trained in health and safety.

Working alone can make you vulnerable. For example, you could be accused of doing something you haven't done. If you can demonstrate that you follow work procedures carefully and are always conscientious in your work, you and those you have to report to will be confident that you have done your job properly.

You read earlier that it is your responsibility to give your team information about what you will be doing, where and when. This is particularly important when you are working alone. It means you can be traced if you get lost, your car breaks down, you don't turn up for an appointment or you are late arriving back at work.

These are just a few examples of the difficulties faced by lone workers. A useful checklist for reducing or preventing them is:

- be trained for the situations you may have to face
- follow work procedures at all times
- be able to make contact with your team or supervisor, e.g. carry a mobile phone or a pager
- never be afraid to ask how to deal with a situation.

DEVELOP GOOD WORK PRACTICE 5.2.2

ACTIVITY 49

1 Talk to your colleagues about difficulties they have experienced when working on their own. Jot down how they coped with any problems

_____

_____

_____

_____

_____

2 Read your workplace's procedures for lone working. Make notes on how it affects your work

_____

_____

_____

_____

_____

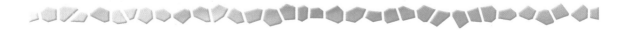

6 Understanding how to apply the care values

In Chapter 1 you learnt about the values of care and how, by using them in your work, you show your service users that you value them. This chapter aims to build on that learning and explain how you can help your service users improve and maintain their value of themselves. It aims to develop your understanding of <u>discrimination</u> and the importance of working in an anti-discriminatory way. It also explores how to cope with the struggles of living and working with other people.

Successful completion of the activities in this chapter will enable you to demonstrate your understanding of the Foundation Standard 'Understand how to apply the value base of care'. It will also give you an opportunity to develop evidence for key skills unit Communication at level I.

What is covered in this chapter?

This chapter contributes to the knowledge and understanding you need for the following NVQ Care units:

O1 : Foster people's equality, diversity and rights

CL1 : Promote effective communication and relationships

CL2 : Promote communication with individuals where there are communication differences

W2 : Contribute to the ongoing support of clients and those who are familiar to them

W3 : Support individuals experiencing a change in their care requirements and provision

Z5 : Enable clients to maintain their mobility and make journeys and visits

Z8 : Support individuals when they are distressed

Z13 : Enable clients to participate in recreation and leisure activities

6.1 EMPOWERMENT

What values are missing from the care given to the following people?

- Molly, who lives in a nursing home and has to eat at the times set by the kitchen team
- Doug, who lives in residential care and has no lock on his room or on the bathroom door
- Rashid, whose carers make every effort to help him avoid having to do anything for himself
- Marie, whose care team has been told by her GP to change the timing of her medication
- Ben, who can no longer attend his West Indian church because the wheelchair-friendly taxi service to the church has been withdrawn.

Do you see that the care given to each person does not respect their rights? Molly lacks the right to choose when she wants to eat, Doug the right to privacy and dignity, Rashid the right to be independent, Marie the right to work in partnership with her GP and have her say about her medication, and Ben the right to worship as he thinks he should.

If we don't respect people's rights, we take away their power to control their lives and live as they would choose. Taking away people's power makes them feel worthless and unimportant.

Empowerment, on the other hand, means respecting people's rights by giving them power. Being empowered lets people take control, make choices, retain their individuality and be independent and responsible for themselves. Empowerment increases people's happiness, self-confidence and the value they have for themselves. It makes them feel important and that they are valued by others.

Because empowerment has such positive effects, it is very important that care workers do all they can to help empower service users. The next section looks at how you can empower your service users by developing the way you use the care values in your work.

Empowering your service users

You can empower your service users by involving them in the way you care for them. They have the right to be partners with the care team in deciding what their individual needs are. They have the right to be partners with you in choosing the help they need to stay as independent as possible. They have the right to be involved in the review of their care and to say how it could be improved.

Empowering service users by involving them in their care respects their right to have a 'voice' or to be heard. Giving service users a 'voice' means listening to them, respecting them for what they have to say and, as far as possible, acting on what they want. There is no point encouraging service users to speak up about their needs and express their concerns if what they have to say is not heard and acted on.

Some of your service users will not be able to use their 'voice'. They may:

- be confused
- lack confidence in speaking up for themselves
- be scared of being seen as trouble makers
- have problems communicating.

In cases like these, service users have a right to an 'advocate' to speak on their behalf, e.g. a family member or a representative from a voluntary organisation such as Age Concern. Or it could be you. Your responsibility as a care worker is to recognise when service users need support in speaking up for themselves. If you are not in a position to advocate for them, you should discuss the situation with your supervisor.

For service users and their advocates to have a 'voice' and be respected for what they have to say, they need to be able to speak with authority. To do this, they need up-to-date information about services and how to use them. You have a responsibility to give your service users and their advocates the information they need, using words and expressions they will understand. If you don't have the information yourself, be prepared to find it for them or to refer them on to your supervisor.

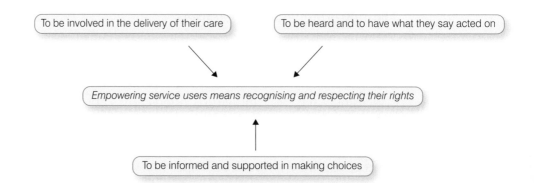

To be involved in the delivery of their care

To be heard and to have what they say acted on

Empowering service users means recognising and respecting their rights

To be informed and supported in making choices

 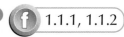 1.1.1, 1.1.2

Think about three of your service users. How can you help them become empowered and how would they benefit from being empowered?

ACTIVITY 50

Service user	How I could help them become empowered	How they would benefit from being empowered
1		
2		

3

_____ _____ _____
_____ _____ _____
_____ _____ _____
_____ _____ _____
_____ _____ _____

▲▲▲

6.2 HELPING SERVICE USERS TO ACHIEVE AND BE FULFILLED

If you listen to people talking about their lives, you will hear them recalling their experiences, their achievements and their disappointments. They might also talk about what they would like to achieve in the future. Their tone of voice and the way they use body language, e.g. their facial expressions would give you an idea about how they feel about their experiences and their dreams for the future.

It goes without saying that our achievements, e.g. building successful relationships, developing new skills and becoming independent give us the greatest pleasure. We get fulfilment – satisfaction and happiness – from our achievements.

Your service users may be elderly, frail or not in good health. Consequently they may believe they have no chance of achieving anything more in their lives. The emotions linked with such an unrewarding future will be the opposite of satisfaction and happiness. It is your responsibility to help them to achieve in whatever ways they can so that they are fulfilled and satisfied now and in the future.

Helping service users maintain contact with family and friends

To be fulfilled, we all need to love and be loved. Keeping in contact with loved ones such as family and friends – and pets – is therefore very important.

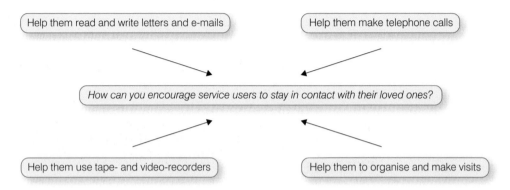

When friends and family come to visit service users, you can help by greeting them politely and making them comfortable, e.g. offer them a cup of tea, give them privacy.

Helping service users develop and maintain social contacts

Belonging to a group and having social contacts is very fulfilling. It gives us the chance to make new friends, to talk about ourselves and our experiences and to feel that we are appreciated.

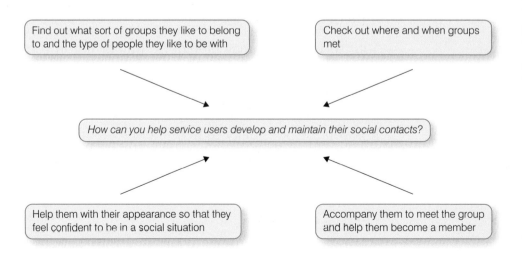

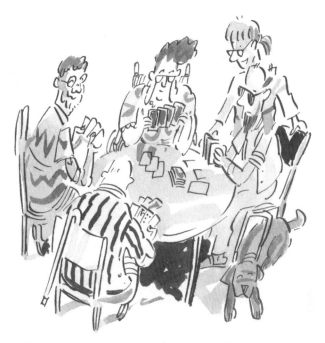

Maintaining social interaction is important for your service users

Helping service users take part in interests and activities

Having interests and taking part in activities are achievements in themselves. They also help us relax, keep our minds active and can help us stay fit.

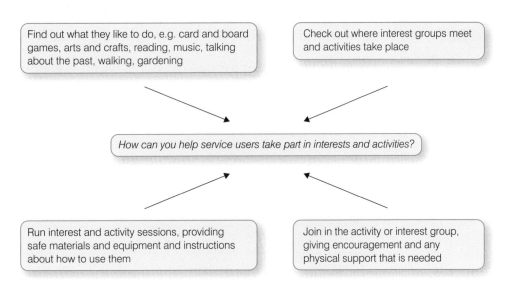

Find out what they like to do, e.g. card and board games, arts and crafts, reading, music, talking about the past, walking, gardening

Check out where interest groups meet and activities take place

How can you help service users take part in interests and activities?

Run interest and activity sessions, providing safe materials and equipment and instructions about how to use them

Join in the activity or interest group, giving encouragement and any physical support that is needed

Helping service users stay mobile

Being able to get around and about independently is a very important achievement. It also helps us keep fit and strong.

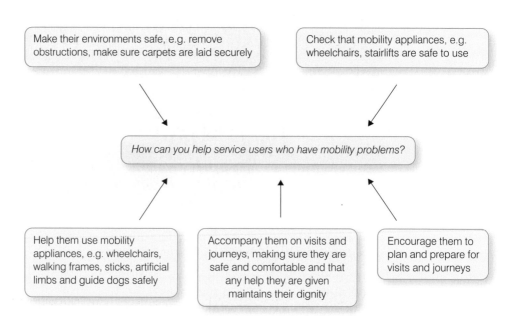

Make their environments safe, e.g. remove obstructions, make sure carpets are laid securely

Check that mobility appliances, e.g. wheelchairs, stairlifts are safe to use

How can you help service users who have mobility problems?

Help them use mobility appliances, e.g. wheelchairs, walking frames, sticks, artificial limbs and guide dogs safely

Accompany them on visits and journeys, making sure they are safe and comfortable and that any help they are given maintains their dignity

Encourage them to plan and prepare for visits and journeys

DEVELOP GOOD WORK PRACTICE   1.2.1

ACTIVITY 51

Talk to two of your service users. Find out what each would like to achieve and how their achievements would make them feel.

Write an action plan for one of your service users describing how you could help him or her to achieve and feel fulfilled.

6.3 THE CONSTRAINTS AND CONFLICTS OF LIVING AND WORKING WITH OTHERS

Constraints are factors that limit what you can do. Conflicts result from disagreements and differences of opinion between people. In this section you will be looking at how to cope with the constraints and conflicts that occur when people are living and working together.

Living with others

It can be very difficult living with other people. You may have experienced conflicts at home because of people not clearing up after themselves, not being able to watch the TV programmes you like or someone hogging the bathroom or telephone! It isn't always easy to live together in peace and harmony.

All this makes for conflict and doesn't sound too much like happy families, does it?

You can play a very important part in helping service users live together happily by being a role model to them. By using the care values in your work, you will be demonstrating your respect for service users':

- rights to privacy and confidentiality of their personal affairs
- rights to express their views and beliefs (in a considerate way)
- rights to safety, protection and freedom from abuse.

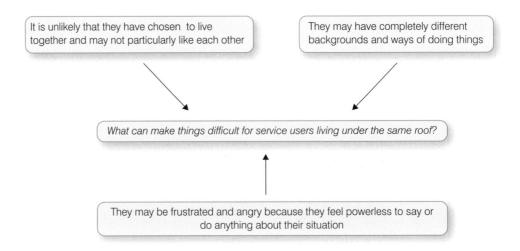

It is unlikely that they have chosen to live together and may not particularly like each other

They may have completely different backgrounds and ways of doing things

What can make things difficult for service users living under the same roof?

They may be frustrated and angry because they feel powerless to say or do anything about their situation

Behaviour that respects people's rights builds good relationships and a happy living environment. In addition, respecting people's individuality and diverse (different) backgrounds and showing that you value everybody equally also makes for friendships and peaceful living.

Some service users have difficulty communicating. This can cause relationship problems. They may speak a different language or have lost the ability to hold a conversation. They may have a hearing loss. They may have a disability and can't use speech or body language, or a sight problem and can't see other people's body language. The way that you show you value their communications sets an example to other service users. In the same way that service users have a right to be 'heard', they have a responsibility to support others in expressing themselves. Good communication makes for good relationships and conflict-free living.

Apart from setting a good example as you do your work, you may sometimes find yourself trying to sort out conflicts. As you become more experienced in your job you will develop the skill of dealing with delicate situations. In the meantime, call upon the judgement of colleagues or your supervisor if situations get difficult.

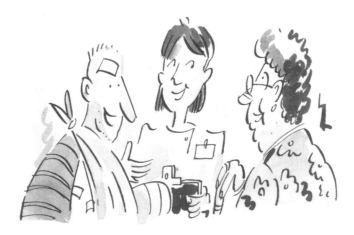

Good communication makes everybody happy

What do you think? 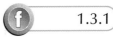 1.3.1

ACTIVITY 52

What problems do you think your service users have living with each other?

Discuss your thoughts with your supervisor and make notes on how you can help prevent or deal with problems created by people living together.

Working with others

Service users are assessed to find out what care they want and need. A 'care package' consists of the services that are used to meet their wants and needs. A 'care plan' describes how and by whom the care package is delivered.

As a care worker, the most important part of your job is to work with service users to help meet their care needs. To do this you must follow their care plans and deliver part of the care package. Others who are involved in delivering care packages are your workplace colleagues, other organisations that provide care services and, of course, service users' families and friends.

In a perfect world, delivering the care package would be simple and straightforward – everybody involved would just follow the care plan. But service users' needs and circumstances change. For example they may lose the ability to get around independently, they may need different medication. This means that care plans and care packages have to be altered.

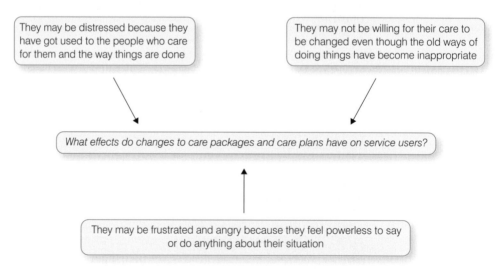

You can help service users at these times by using the care values to empower them:

- use your communication skills to explain why their care needs to change

- give them a 'voice' and encourage them to say how they would choose to be cared for
- make sure that they feel involved in decisions made about changes to their care.

Keep your supervisor informed about their feelings and preferences for care. Every effort will be made to build feelings and preferences into the revised care plan.

CHECK YOUR UNDERSTANDING

 1.3.2

ACTIVITY 53

CASE STUDY: *Irwin*

Irwin is gradually losing his ability to get around on his own and he now needs to wear incontinence pads during the day as well as at night. He is very frustrated with himself and resents the fact that the care he receives has to change.

List ways you could work with Irwin to help him come to terms with his changing care needs.

6.4 ANTI-DISCRIMINATORY PRACTICE

Can you see anything wrong with the following statements?

- the amputee
- the aggressive patient
- the disabled cook
- the confused service user.

The problem with talking about people like this is that they are being labelled according to one of their characteristics. All their other qualities seem to be unimportant. Labelling people makes them feel 'just a number' and that everything else about them is not worth talking about.

Stereotyping is to do with judging people according to characteristics such as their age, ability, health, sex, sexual preference, appearance and religion. Many people believe that everyone who shares a characteristic will be the same in every other way. But while one elderly person may be confused, it is far from the truth that all elderly people are confused. Stereotyping or 'lumping' people together like this and assuming they are all the same doesn't show respect for their individuality.

Discrimination means behaving in an unfair way towards a person because of the way we have judged them. Discrimination or unfair treatment can take many forms. For example:

- older people are often not asked for their opinion because they are considered 'past it', despite their wisdom and understanding
- people with physical disabilities are often treated as being dim-witted even though it may be only their legs that don't work
- people with mental health problems are often treated with fear and unfriendliness when perhaps they are just anxious and don't behave in an expected way.

Being discriminated against can make people feel unimportant, worthless, frustrated and angry. It can result in them not having the same opportunities at school or in getting a job. Discrimination does not respect people's rights.

<u>Oppression</u> is discrimination that is cruel and bullying. People who practise oppression are usually more powerful than those they oppress. They dominate and abuse them. Being oppressed makes people feel crushed and without hope. Oppression doesn't respect rights and it takes away dignity.

So, labelling, stereotyping, discrimination and oppression all go against the values of care. Your responsibility as a care worker is to ensure that your service users are treated in an anti-discriminatory, anti-oppressive way.

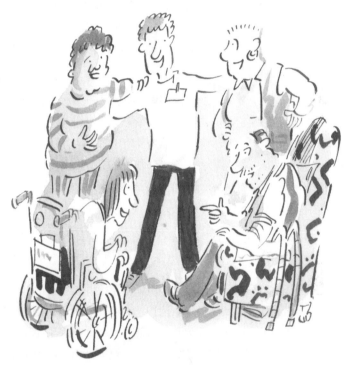

Everyone shares the same thoughts and feelings

Overcoming discrimination

Do you discriminate against service users? For example, do you:

- 'lump' them together and treat them all the same? – for example, they are all elderly so they must all enjoy playing bingo or want everything done for them …

- use words and laugh at jokes that are rude and hurtful because they are ageist (to do with age), sexist, racist or about people with disabilities?

Admitting that you do discriminate will help you challenge your behaviour and improve the way you work with service users. It will also put you in a better position to recognise and challenge other people's discriminatory behaviour.

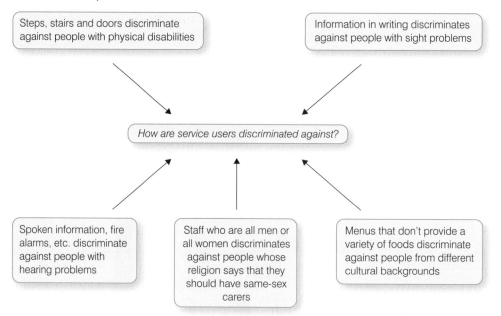

You have a responsibility to challenge anything that makes life unfair for service users. Talk to the people who are responsible for ensuring that the Disability Discrimination Act 1995, the Race Relations Act 1976 and the Sex Discrimination Act 1975 are complied with.

Not all discrimination is covered by laws. If you hear service users being called names, being bullied because of their views and beliefs or being treated unfairly in any way, support them by challenging the person concerned. If you are not confident enough to make a challenge, get help from a colleague or your supervisor.

Service users are vulnerable and need support. By playing your part in overcoming discrimination you will be protecting their rights to fair treatment and respect for their individuality, self-worth, dignity, safety and freedom from abuse.

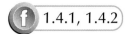

ACTIVITY 54

Complete the table to show that you understand how to behave in an anti-discriminatory way and why this is important.

Service users	How the service user might be discriminated against	How you could challenge discrimination against the service user	Why it is important to challenge discrimination against the service user
Mrs A who has mobility problems			
Mr B who has a sight impairment			

7 Understanding how to communicate effectively

As you read in Chapter 1, care workers need to be able to communicate effectively and appropriately with service users, colleagues and other people they come across in their day-to-day work. This chapter aims to help you build on your communication skills and show you how you can support service users in their communications with you.

Successful completion of the activities in this chapter will enable you to demonstrate your understanding of the Foundation Standard *Communicate effectively*. It will also give you an opportunity to develop evidence for key skills unit Communication at level 1.

7.1 ENCOURAGING SERVICE USERS TO COMMUNICATE WITH YOU

Service users have a right to be heard but may find it difficult to communicate. They may speak another language, have a sight or hearing loss, be ill or distressed. However, to do your job properly you need to know how they feel, what they want and need and if they have any concerns. So you need them to communicate with you.

How you encourage service users to communicate will depend on their specific difficulties. Find out what the problems are. Good sources of information are the service users themselves (the experts), their family and friends, their records and other people who work with them. When you understand their problems you can help them communicate in the way they choose, e.g. writing, sign language, pictures, interpreters. You will also realise the importance of making sure that hearing aids, glasses and so on are in good order.

Whatever service users' difficulties are, your behaviour is important in encouraging them to communicate with you.

How to encourage communication	How to put people off communicating with you
Speak clearly to make yourself understood	Mutter and mumble
Use words and expressions that people understand	Use confusing technical terms and slang
Talk at a speed and volume that people can cope with	Talk too quickly, too quietly or too loudly
Use an appropriate tone of voice	Sound cheerful when you should sound sad
Use body language that shows you are interested and paying attention	Look bored and anxious to escape
Use forms of communication that people prefer, e.g. writing and pictures	Stick to communication methods you know best
Help people to communicate with each other	Don't offer any support
Respect people's preferences and expectations about how to communicate with them	Talk to everybody in the same way, regardless of their age, sex and background

How good are you at encouraging service users to communicate?

7.2 USING LISTENING SKILLS TO ENCOURAGE COMMUNICATION

There is little point respecting service users' right to have a voice and encouraging them to communicate with you if you don't listen to what they tell you! For this reason it is important that you develop your listening skills.

> *CASE STUDY: Mr S*
>
> *Mr S used to be very chatty but recently has become quiet, preferring to sit on his own; and he looks troubled.*

Your supervisor has asked you to spend some time with Mr S, to find out what is troubling him. How would you encourage Mr S to talk to you about the way he feels?

You already know that appropriate body language shows you are paying attention and are interested in what you are being told. So, as a good listener you would:

- look at Mr S as you and he chat together
- sit in a relaxed position, leaning slightly forward to help you concentrate on what he tells you
- change your tone of voice and the expression on your face to imitate his feelings
- nod your head and make encouraging noises like 'yes' and 'mmm'.

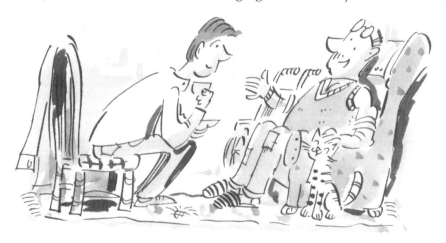

A good listener makes service users feel comfortable in expressing their feelings and concerns

Good listeners do more than just hear words and recognise feelings. They also 'read between the lines' or 'hear' what isn't said. In this way they get a full understanding of what is being communicated.

> *Mr S tells you that his daughter is having problems at home and doesn't have time to visit him any more.*

'Reading between the lines', what do you think Mr S is saying? Maybe that in addition to being worried about his daughter, he is missing her visits and becoming lonely and depressed?

As a good listener you will pick up on things that aren't actually said but it is important to check that your understanding is correct. Don't assume that what you have 'heard' is correct. The way we 'hear' things can change depending on the way we feel. For example, do you hear things in the same way when you are busy and stressed as when you are relaxed and have lots of time to spare? Check your understanding by asking questions that give service users the chance to express themselves more clearly.

The point about being a good listener is that, if you show interest and try to understand what you are being told, your service users will feel valued and be encouraged to tell you more. And the more you know, the better you will be able work with them and do your job.

DEVELOP GOOD WORK PRACTICE

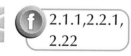 2.1.1, 2.2.1, 2.22

ACTIVITY 55

1 Observe the way your colleagues use communication and listening skills to encourage service users to communicate with them. List the methods that are most successful

2 Ask your supervisor for feedback on your listening skills. Make a list of the skills you use now and another list of those you need to develop

Listening skills I use now	Listening skills I need to develop

7.3 USING PHYSICAL CONTACT TO ENCOURAGE COMMUNICATION

As well as using words, body language and listening skills to encourage communication, we can also use touch (physical contact). Much of your care work involves the use of touch, for example when you give:

- emotional support, e.g. stroking a hand, giving a hug
- physical support and protection, e.g. guiding and supporting those with poor sight or mobility problems
- signalling your presence to a deaf service user by a touch on the shoulder
- support with day-to-day living activities, e.g. eating and drinking, bathing, using the toilet, getting dressed, shaving.

Supporting service users in these ways shows that you value them and encourages them to communicate with you. But not everybody is comfortable being touched. How would you feel if you had to have your bottom wiped by someone you didn't know very well? How would you feel if your religion said that only close relatives were allowed to touch you, or if you were abused as a child and you have to be bathed and undressed by someone else? Uncomfortable? Embarrassed? Shamed? Angry?

Feelings like this inhibit (prevent) communication between people. So when you give care that involves touching service users it is important that:

- you have their permission
- they are completely at ease with everything you do
- you use words and body language that will help them keep their dignity and feel confident, safe and secure.

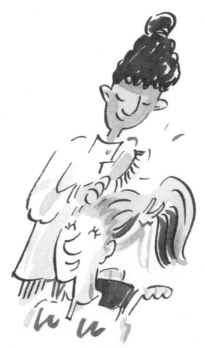

Touch is an important method of communication

Communication by touch is especially important for service users who have problems seeing and hearing. Signing through touch can help deaf people express themselves and 'hear' others; and vibrating equipment and raised symbols such as braille are useful for communicating information to service users who cannot see. Make it your responsibility to learn how each of your service users prefers to communicate and how to get help, e.g. signers, training.

CHECK YOUR UNDERSTANDING

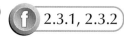 2.3.1, 2.3.2

ACTIVITY 56

Write an anonymous case study of one of your service users that describes:

- the physical contact you have with them and how you use it to encourage them to communicate with you
- when and why you wouldn't use physical contact with them.

7.4 COMMUNICATION BARRIERS AND CHALLENGING BEHAVIOUR

Communication barriers

Communication is difficult when there are barriers that prevent people expressing themselves or being seen, heard or understood.

> **CASE STUDY: Grace**
>
> *Grace is at the Health Centre with her residential care worker, waiting to see the doctor. She is very worried about her health. The waiting room is hot, stuffy and gloomy. It's also noisy because of telephones, the traffic outside and chatter from the office.*
> *The receptionist calls Grace to the desk and asks her a string of questions, using lots of medical expressions. The receptionist is from another country – neither Grace nor her care worker recognise the accent – and seems to be quite stressed.*

Do you think that the receptionist would succeed in obtaining the information she needs from Grace? Not likely – the situation is loaded with communication barriers!

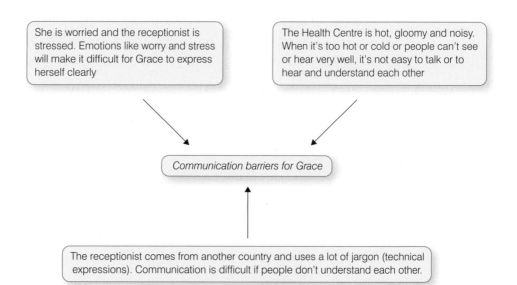

She is worried and the receptionist is stressed. Emotions like worry and stress will make it difficult for Grace to express herself clearly

The Health Centre is hot, gloomy and noisy. When it's too hot or cold or people can't see or hear very well, it's not easy to talk or to hear and understand each other

Communication barriers for Grace

The receptionist comes from another country and uses a lot of jargon (technical expressions). Communication is difficult if people don't understand each other.

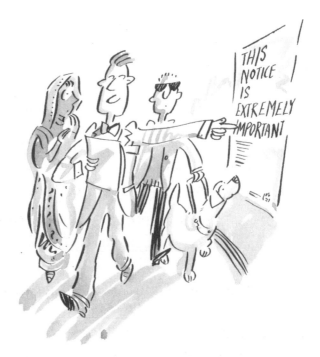

Be aware of the communication barriers that exist

This sort of situation is quite common so it's no wonder that people misunderstand each other and that there are breakdowns in communication. But you need your service users to communicate with you, so it is your responsibility to:

- be alert to what makes it difficult for them to communicate
- play your part in making things easier for them – breaking down the barriers.

Don't forget that the problem could be you! Does the way you behave encourage communication? Do you adapt the way you communicate to meet the needs of service users who are deaf, blind or have particular disabilities?

Ways that you can help break down communicating barriers

Communication barriers experienced by service users	How you can help
Emotional difficulties, e.g. stress, worry	Be patient, show your concern, use your listening skills
Language differences	Think about using an interpreter or translator or make an effort to learn their language
Jargon, slang or accents that are difficult to understand	Explain what the words and expressions mean or, better still, use alternatives that will be understood
An uncomfortable environment and sensory impairments	Find out how you can improve things and check that hearing aids and glasses are in working order

DEVELOP GOOD WORK PRACTICE 2.4.1

ACTIVITY 57

Talk to two or three service users about difficulties they have communicating with you, your colleagues and their friends and family. Jot down what they tell you and make notes on how you can help break down these barriers.

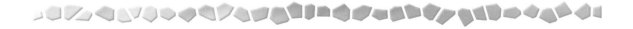

Dealing with challenging behaviour

Challenging behaviour can be verbal, e.g. insulting, shouting and swearing. It can also be physical, e.g. aggression, violence and self-harming. But whether it is spoken or physical, it is upsetting and disruptive. More importantly, it fails to show respect for others. Service users – and care workers – have a right to be respected.

Service users can behave in challenging ways for a number of reasons. They may:

- be distressed because of bad news
- be stressed because of noise or relationship problems
- have a low opinion of themselves because they've lost their independence
- not recognise that their behaviour is 'out of line' because they are confused or on medication that has changed their behaviour.

If you've ever been in a situation that has caused you to lose your temper, you'll know how difficult it is at the time to talk and listen in a sensible and reasonable way. As a care worker, you have a responsibility to try to prevent situations becoming explosive through the use of effective communication.

It is important to respect service users' right to choose how to behave but it is equally important that service users behave in ways that show respect for others. Find out from your colleagues which service users can become disruptive and what can trigger changes in their behaviour.

If things do get out of hand and behaviour becomes upsetting, try to calm things down. Use words, body language and a tone of voice that are soothing and reassuring. But if things become violent and unsafe, your priority is to get yourself and others out of danger and to call for help. Don't try to deal with situations like this until you have more experience.

Your workplace will have procedures that describe how to deal with incidents of challenging behaviour, including how you should report and record them. There are training courses you can attend that will help

you develop the skills needed for dealing with challenging behaviour.
Find out what they are.

DEVELOP GOOD WORK PRACTICE 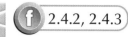 2.4.2, 2.4.3

ACTIVITY 58

1 Find out from your colleagues how they communicate with service
users who become disruptive.

2 Read your workplace's procedure for dealing with violent behaviour
and jot down the main points.

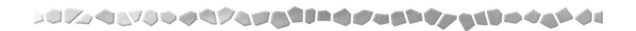

7.5 PRODUCING RECORDS AND REPORTS

Records and reports you use or contribute to

In your caring role, you will be given information from service users,
their family and friends, your colleagues and manager, people from other
care organisations, health and social care professionals – the list is
endless! In addition to being given information, you may have to give
information to others.

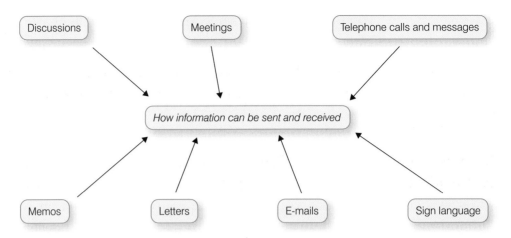

You already know how important the spoken word, body language and listening skills are for effective communication (sending and receiving information). This section looks at the importance of written communication in sending and receiving information.

Think for a moment about the sort of written information that you use or contribute to during your day-to-day work. Your list might include care plans and records, workplace policies and procedures, accident reports, health and safety instructions, timesheets and telephone messages.

The written information you use is important because it tells how to do your job properly. For example:

- care plans describe the package of care that has been agreed for a service user and your role in delivering that care
- workplace procedures describe how you must carry out work activities.

The written information you contribute to is equally important because it keeps other people informed about service users and helps them to do their job. For example:

- accident records inform families, your colleagues and health professionals about injuries to service users; they also inform your employer and maintenance staff about health and safety hazards that need to be dealt with
- daily reports keep colleagues up-to-date about individual service users.

CHECK YOUR UNDERSTANDING

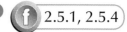 2.5.1, 2.5.4

Complete the table to show your understanding of the purpose of records and reports that you use or contribute to and who might want or need to read them.

Records or reports I use/contribute to	Purpose of these records and reports	Who might want or need to see these records and reports

How should you write records and reports?

It is extremely important that written information is readable and understandable.

Telephone message

While you were out ...

Mrs H rang the bell isn't working today there's a chap coming

Bill

Although we can read what Bill has said, is it understandable? Did Mrs. H use the 'phone to ring in to work – or did she ring the bell? Is it Mrs. H or the bell that isn't working? Is the chap coming today, is Mrs. B not working today or is it the bell that's not working today? And when is 'today'? – there's no date. All very confusing! Whenever you take a message, make sure it is written down so that someone else can understand it.

Written information must also be relevant and to the point, i.e. it must only include what is important.

Mr J didn't eat much breakfast this morning. He ate some of the egg but none of the bread and he left his cup of tea on the bedside table. It was cold. When I went to collect his tray he was watching the t.v. There was a programme on about gardening and he told me he used to enjoy working on his allotment. He used to grow his own vegetables and sell them when he had too many for his own use.
P. White 1st April 10 am

This message is understandable, but it rambles on and much of what is said isn't relevant and important.

Finally, written information must contain only facts that can be checked. Other people may need to read what you have written or that somebody else has written on your behalf. So you need to be sure that your records and reports are accurate.

What do you think is wrong with this daily report?

Dorothy Brown was a bit of a pain this evening. She had a right old moan at me when I took her in her bedtime drink. She's got another bruise on her arm. Fallen over again I suppose.
Wendy, 1 April 9pm

First of all, how do you think Dorothy would feel if she discovered she'd been described as a 'bit of a pain' and having 'had a right old moan'? Annoyed? Insulted? Remarks like these are subjective – they are one person's point of view and not how somebody else might describe Dorothy. They aren't necessarily true, can't be checked and so shouldn't have been put down in writing.

Secondly, had Dorothy really fallen over? This remark may well be true and it can be checked. But it shouldn't be written down until it has been checked and proved to be true.

The daily report about Dorothy should have been written like this:

Dorothy Brown wasn't very happy this evening, especially when I gave her some hot milk. She has a bruise on her arm. This needs investigating please.
Wendy, 1 April 9pm

To sum up, records and reports that you write (that someone else writes on your behalf) should be:

- easy to read
- easy to understand
- to the point
- relevant
- factual
- checkable.

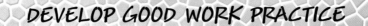 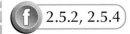

DEVELOP GOOD WORK PRACTICE (f) 2.5.2, 2.5.4

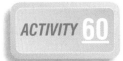

ACTIVITY 60 Talk with your supervisor about the records and reports that you write (or that someone writes on your behalf). Tick the boxes to show which written communication skills you are good at and which skills you need to improve on.

Written communication skills	Skills I am good at	Skills I need to improve
My writing is easy to read	☐	☐
Records and reports that I write are easy to understand	☐	☐
Records and reports that I write are to the point	☐	☐
Records and reports that I write include only relevant information	☐	☐
Records and reports that I write include only factual information	☐	☐
Records and reports that I write include information that can be checked	☐	☐

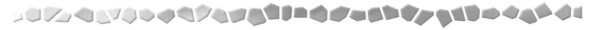

Just about everybody needs to improve their written communication skills! Find out about courses you could enrol on that will help you improve your report-writing skills.

Records, reports and confidentiality

The Data Protection Act 1998 is in place to make sure that the personal information in written records and reports is protected. Protecting someone's personal information shows respect for their right to privacy. It also prevents them from being harmed by misuse of their personal information.

Your workplace obeys the Data Protection Act by having policies and procedures that describe which records and reports are to be protected and how. As a general rule, anything that contains sensitive information about service users should be protected and kept confidential.

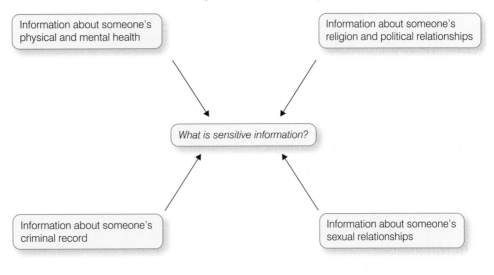

CASE STUDY: *Ivor*

Ivor had a nervous breakdown in his fifties which led to him becoming homeless, getting into trouble with the law and spending a period of time in prison. He is now 73 and living in residential care.

How do you think Ivor would be affected if this information became a subject of gossip in the residential home? He might feel vulnerable and betrayed and would think twice before telling anybody anything about himself. He might be treated with suspicion or rejected by the other residents and become isolated and lonely.

You have a responsibility to maintain the confidentiality of service users' personal information. This means not letting other people read their records and reports unless:

- they have been given permission by the service user
- they have a right or they need to know the information, e.g. information about health risks or abuse will need to be shared with other health and care organisations.

Your workplace policies and procedures will tell you who you can share information with and under what conditions.

Maintaining the confidentiality of records and reports means taking precautions to make sure that nobody can:

- overhear what service users tell you – respect their privacy and have discussions behind closed doors
- oversee what you write in records and reports – if you are using a computer, make sure that the monitor is angled so that others can't see what you are typing.

Records and reports should be looked after carefully – don't leave them lying around. And they should be stored securely in locked filing cabinets or computer files that can only be opened by people with a secure password.

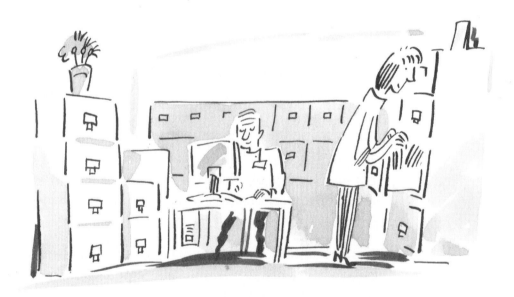

Records and reports should be stored appropriately in order to protect your service users' confidentiality

CHECK YOUR UNDERSTANDING 2.5.3

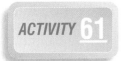

For Activity 59 you made a list of records and reports you write or contribute to in your day-to-day work. List which of these documents needs to be kept confidential and say why and how they are protected.

Records and reports that must be kept confidential	Why they must be kept confidential	How they are kept confidential

8 Understanding how to develop as a worker

To improve the way you work, increase your chances of promotion and stay fulfilled in your job, you need to continually develop your knowledge and understanding of care work, learn new skills, stay up-to-date with care issues and look after yourself physically and emotionally. The aim of this chapter is to raise your awareness of your learning needs and encourage you to take responsibility for your development, health and safety. It also builds on what you have learnt about effective communication, the effects of the service setting on you as a worker and how to maintain safety at work.

Successful completion of the activities in this chapter will enable you to demonstrate your understanding of the Foundation Standard *Develop as a worker*. It will also give you an opportunity to develop evidence for key skills unit Communication at level 1.

What is covered in this chapter?

This chapter contributes to the knowledge and understanding you need for the following NVQ Care units:
CU1 : Promote, monitor and maintain health, safety and security in the workplace
CU3 : Monitor and maintain the cleanliness of environments
CU4 : Support and control visitors to services and facilities
CU10 : Contribute to the effectiveness of work teams

8.1 LEARNING ON AND OFF THE JOB

Take a few minutes to think about everything you've learned while you have been working in care. Include all the hands-on caring tasks as well as the behind-the-scenes chores like housework, answering the phone, paper work and the meetings and discussions you attend.

You will probably be quite surprised at how clever you are! Care work is multiskilled and care workers have to have a wide knowledge and understanding.

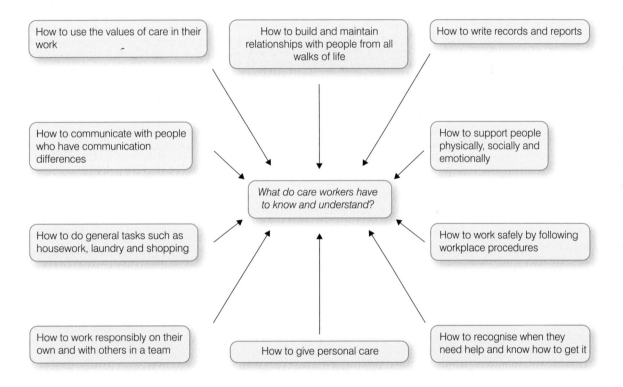

How did you learn all that you know now? Much of what you know will have been learned by 'shadowing' a senior worker to see how they did things and then having a go yourself. You might have attended some in-house training sessions such as first aid and moving and handling. Doing things yourself – 'hands on' learning – is a good way to develop the skills you need for your work.

Listening and reading are also good ways to learn about and improve the way you do your job. At induction, your supervisor or manager might have talked to you about the care values and how to meet the needs of individual service users. They will have told you about workplace policies and procedures, and records and reports you have to use and write. And of course reading this book and doing the activities has given you the opportunity to improve and provide evidence for your learning about what makes for good care practice.

How can you continue to learn and improve your performance so that you become valued and respected by everyone you work with? The answer is to:

- ask your colleagues for feedback on your current performance and how you can improve the way you work
- think about your own performance and identify your strengths and weaknesses.

Then, armed with feedback from your colleagues and your own identification of your learning needs, check out and take advantage of all the learning opportunities available to you. You could, for example:

- continue to watch and listen to your colleagues – their experience is invaluable and something you should take advantage of
- attend training sessions that your supervisor or manager organises for you
- read specialist care magazines and journals – these will keep you informed about your job role and up-to-date on issues to do with caring
- watch educational TV programmes and videos
- check out care-related Internet websites – these will also keep you up-to-date on a wide variety of care topics
- enrol on a course at your local college – you could, for example, learn about areas of care that are quite new to you or brush up your communication skills

- enrol on a care-related Internet course – the advantage of these courses is that you can study at a time that is best for you
- join a voluntary group or sports team, help run Cubs or Brownies, get together with a crowd of friends and take part in pub quizzes – being with other people in situations like this will help you develop your teamwork skills.

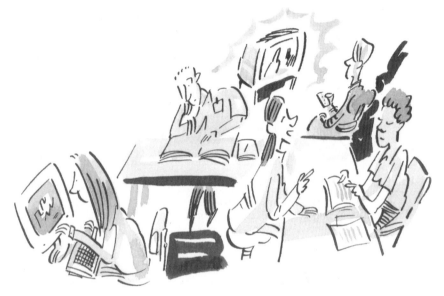

There are numerous ways to improve your knowledge

Don't just go for the learning opportunities that are planned for you at work. Check out opportunities for yourself, ones that you know you will enjoy. You learn more when it is fun. Apart from making you better at your job and more likely to get promotion, improving your learning will earn you respect from others and increase your self-confidence and self-esteem.

What do you think?

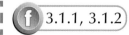 3.1.1, 3.1.2

ACTIVITY 62

Complete the table about three things you have learned in your job. How did you prepare for doing the learning? Did you send off for a college prospectus or was it organised for you at work? Did you have to organise child care, take time off work or change your shift? Did you have to do any preparatory reading?

How did you do the learning? Did you learn by observation, by attending a training course, by going to college, by reading?

How do you think your learning has changed the way you do your work?

What I have learned in my job	How I prepared for the learning	How I did the learning	How my learning has changed the way I do my work

You and your supervisor

You read earlier about the importance of discussing your performance at work with your colleagues. You also read about the need to reflect on your strengths and weaknesses so that you can identify for yourself where you need to make improvements. Your supervisor's main role is to work with you, both to help you improve the way you do your job and also to support you in your personal development.

Your supervisor is a trusted colleague. It is your supervisor's role to give you feedback on your performance on a regular, daily basis; to discuss your work with you on a weekly or monthly basis; and to carry out appraisals with you, probably once or twice a year. The purpose of feedback, discussions and appraisals is to:

- discuss how well you think you are doing your job
- discuss how you think you can improve the way you do things, e.g. by improving your learning and skills or suggesting how your team might change the way it works
- discuss how your supervisor thinks you can improve the way you do things – be open to feedback and check your understanding of what you are told; if you're not confident that you can change in the way you are asked, be honest about how you feel and discuss alternatives
- help you deal with problems that affect your work, e.g. distressing work procedures, relationship problems, your personal life and your health
- plan for your future development – you can use this plan to monitor your improvement and development.

Your supervisor is there to guide and advise you. Welcome their comments and act on what they tell you.

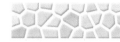 **DEVELOP GOOD WORK PRACTICE** 3.1.3

ACTIVITY 63

Think of two or three recent occasions when you have discussed your work with your supervisor. Note down what you talked about and how your work performance has changed as a result.

_____

_____

_____

_____

_____

_____

_____

_____

_____

_____

_____

_____

_____

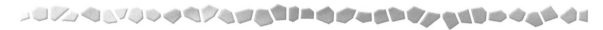

8.2 STAYING SAFE AND HEALTHY

Staying safe

You have read a great deal so far about your responsibilities in protecting the health and safety of the people you work with. This section looks at the risks to your own safety and well-being and how they can be minimised.

You now know that there are laws and regulations to protect you when you are at work. These state that your employer has a responsibility to assess your workplace and the work you do for risks to your safety and to get rid of the risks or reduce them to a minimum.

Workplace risks to safety	Examples of hazards
Obstacles that prevent you moving around safely	Furniture, curled-up rugs, trailing flexes
Faulty gas appliances	Water heaters, cookers, fires
Faulty electric and electronic equipment	Fires, computers, vacuum cleaners, kettles, wheelchairs, hoists, slings
Unsafe conditions	Poor lighting, rotting floorboards, dirt, pests
Hazardous cleaning materials	Toilet cleaners, bleach, disinfectants
Body fluids	Urine, faeces, blood, vomit, mucus
Working alone	Aggressive or threatening people, pets and pests
Moving and handling	Heavy, awkward loads

Hazards like these can cause accidents, first aid incidents and disabilities, e.g. sprains and strains, fractures, scalds and burns, electric shocks and breathing problems. They can cause spread of infection, stress and distress. If you are affected in any of these ways, you will not be able to do your job properly, you may have to take time off work or you may never be able to work again.

Because you follow safe working procedures based on your employer's risk assessments, risks to your safety will be kept to an absolute minimum. However, you should always be prepared to respond to fresh and unexpected risks.

Avoid taking unnecessary risks by knowing what you are capable of doing and what your job description says you can do. Only deal with risks that won't affect your safety, don't take chances and don't try to be a hero. If a task you are doing looks as if it might cause an accident or injury, stop immediately and reassess how it should be done. Only continue when you are confident that it is safe for you to do so.

Know what you can't do. Get help from someone who is better able to deal with the risk than you. For example, if a visitor to the workplace is becoming disruptive and you're not sure how to deal with the situation, set off an alarm or use a mobile phone to contact someone more senior than you. Even if you are working alone, remember you are part of a team and are not expected to be experienced at everything and to cope entirely on your own.

Report the risk to your supervisor or manager. If you have to write a report, remember to make it readable, to the point and factual. Your experience may lead to a new work procedure being written.

Your priority is to take care of yourself. By staying safe, you will be able to care for your service users and support the members of your team.

DEVELOP GOOD WORK PRACTICE

 3.2.1

ACTIVITY 64

List three risks to your personal safety at work. What steps should be taken to keep these risks to a minimum?

Risk	Steps required
1	
2	
3	

Staying healthy

Staying healthy means taking care of yourself physically and emotionally. This section looks at how you can look after your physical health by eating well and having enough rest and relaxation.

To do your job well it is important that you eat a healthy, well balanced diet.

Foods that we need for a healthy diet	Why we need these foods in our diet
Foods containing proteins, e.g. meat, fish, milk, eggs, beans, wheat, soya	For growth and repair
Foods containing carbohydrates and fibre, e.g. bread, cereals, pasta, fruit, vegetables	To give us energy and prevent constipation
Foods that contain fat, e.g. meat, cheese, eggs Foods that contain oil, e.g. olive oil, margarine, oily fish such as sardines	To keep us warm and to give us energy
Foods that contain vitamins and minerals, e.g. fruit and vegetables	For general good health

A balanced diet is one that contains enough of these foods to match individual needs. For example, a growing, active child needs more growth, repair and energy foods than a fully grown adult who works at a desk. And a builder working outdoors will need more energy and insulation foods than an office worker. But they all need vitamins and minerals and fibre to keep their bodies in good working order.

If we eat lots of energy foods but don't use much energy in our daily activities, any unused energy is turned into body fat. This is how we become overweight and obese. If you are overweight or obese, you have a greater risk of heart disease and breathing problems. You won't be fit and you could have a poor self-image. Equally importantly, you won't be able do your job properly.

If you don't eat enough of the foods you need, you will become underweight, weak and short of energy. You will have an increased risk of catching infections and suffering 'nutritional deficiency diseases' such as anaemia, soft bones and night blindness. Again, you won't be able to do your job properly.

Although everybody's dietary needs are different, in general you should aim to:

- fill up on energy foods such as bread, potatoes and cereals
- eat plenty of fruit and vegetables
- eat smaller portions of meat, fish, beans and milk, cheese, eggs (dairy foods)
- keep fatty and sugary foods to a minimum as they will make you fat and rot your teeth – think of them as treats!
- drink at least one litre of water every day.

Other foods that cause ill health are salt and alcohol. Too much salt causes high blood pressure and heart disease. Alcohol causes liver disease, relationship problems, traffic accidents and so on.

To be able to do your job properly you also need to have enough rest and relaxation when you are not at work. Rest and relaxation include sleeping and taking part in recreational activities.

Sleep is important because it provides the opportunity for your body to:

- unwind and calm down
- repair itself
- top up its reserves of energy.

If you don't get enough sleep, you will become short-tempered, rundown and sluggish. In other words, you won't be able to do your job properly.

Taking part in recreational activities is good for you, particularly if it means you get more exercise.

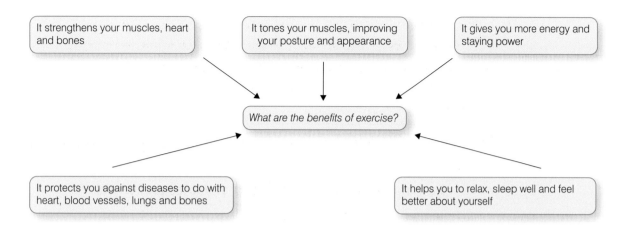

It strengthens your muscles, heart and bones

It tones your muscles, improving your posture and appearance

It gives you more energy and staying power

What are the benefits of exercise?

It protects you against diseases to do with heart, blood vessels, lungs and bones

It helps you to relax, sleep well and feel better about yourself

Other forms of recreational activities include reading, watching the television, going shopping or for a drink with your friends and playing with the children. In other words, they are anything that you enjoy doing, both on your own and with other people, and that, by recharging your batteries, enables you to do your job properly.

What do you think?

 3.2.2

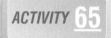

Keep a diary for a week in which you note down:

- what you eat every day
- how much sleep you get every day
- what you do for relaxation every day.

At the end of the week write a few sentences that sum up how healthy you think your lifestyle is.

_____

_____

_____

_____

_____

_____

_____

_____

Write yourself an action plan including how, why and when you should make changes to your lifestyle.

_____

_____

_____

_____

_____

_____

_____

_____

_____

_____

_____

_____

_____

_____

_____

_____

_____

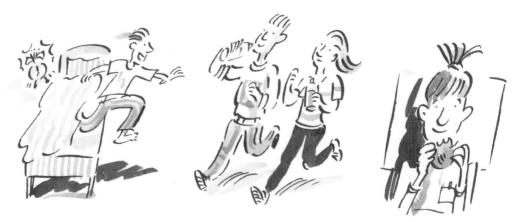

Plenty of sleep, exercise and a balanced diet are key ingredients to staying healthy

Staying stress-free

Stress can be good in small doses. It can stimulate us to work harder and deal with situations that can be quite challenging, such as taking faulty goods back to a shop. But when we can't escape from stressful circumstances, such as when we get stuck in a traffic jam and are going to be late for an appointment, when we just don't get on with a colleague or service user, or when the bills are piling up and there's no chance of being able to pay them, stress can be very damaging to our health.

Think about times when you have been 'stressed out'. How did you feel? Stress affects different people in different emotional ways.

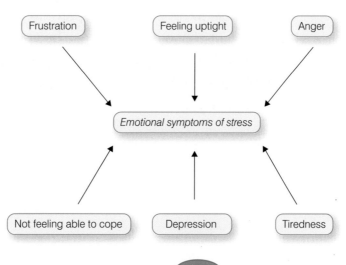

Stress also affects different people in different physical ways.

Headaches and tense muscles

Asthma

Cold sores, coughs and colds

Physical symptoms of stress

Ulcers

Problems with sleeping

High blood pressure

You need to know how to deal with stress before it affects your health. Again, everyone is different, but the following ideas might work for you:

- do something active. Stress produces energy. Use it up by going for a run, doing some exercise, making a cup of tea
- tell someone how you feel. It helps to talk and get things off your chest
- do something to relax. Having a bath, lighting an aromatherapy candle and practising yoga are peaceful and calming things to do

If you are stressed to the point where your health begins to suffer, you won't be able to do your job properly. In such a situation, you should talk with your supervisor. They may be able to help or, if not, to refer you on to others who can, such as your GP, therapists, counsellors, telephone helplines and voluntary organisations who specialise in stress-related problems.

CHECK YOUR UNDERSTANDING

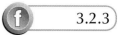

3.2.3

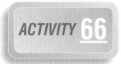

Complete the table to check your understanding of stress.

Factors that cause me to get stressed	The effects that stress has on me	How I can deal with my stress

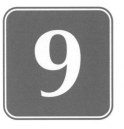

9 Understanding how to recognise and respond to abuse and neglect

As a care worker, you need to be able to recognise if service users are being abused or neglected and whether they are neglecting themselves. You also need to know how to deal with abuse and neglect. This chapter aims to help you protect service users by giving you an understanding of the signs and symptoms of abuse and neglect and of how to respond to situations where you think abuse and neglect may be taking place. It builds on what you have learnt about the principles of care, effective communication and your role as a worker.

Successful completion of the activities in this chapter will enable you to demonstrate your understanding of the Foundation Standard *Recognise and respond to abuse and neglect*. It will also give you an opportunity to develop evidence for key skills unit Communication at level 1.

What is covered in this chapter?

This chapter contributes to the knowledge and understanding you need for the following NVQ Care units:

O1 : Foster people's equality, diversity and rights

Z1 : Contribute to the protection of individuals from abuse

Z8 : Support individuals when they are distressed

9.1 RECOGNISING ABUSE

Abuse is cruel behaviour. It disempowers people and has distressing, disturbing and long-lasting effects on physical and emotional health and well-being. It is usually carried out on purpose by the abuser so that they can be seen to be powerful and 'in charge'.

Service users are particularly vulnerable to abuse because they are often weak and defenceless. You have only to read the papers and watch the television to realise how frequently service user groups such as elderly people and children are taken advantage of and mistreated.

It is your responsibility to protect service users from abuse. You can rest assured that you won't be guilty of abusive behaviour if you always use the care values in your work. Any activity that does not involve you using the values of care is likely to be abusive.

Physical abuse

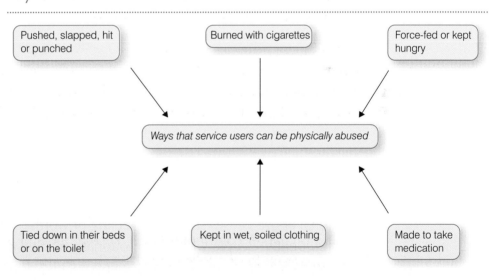

Pushed, slapped, hit or punched

Burned with cigarettes

Force-fed or kept hungry

Ways that service users can be physically abused

Tied down in their beds or on the toilet

Kept in wet, soiled clothing

Made to take medication

Physical abuse causes broken bones, bruises, finger marks, restraint marks, sores, burns and blisters and changes in behaviour such as fear, withdrawal and depression. It denies service users their rights to choice, safety and protection. It also takes away their dignity and shows them no respect.

Sexual abuse

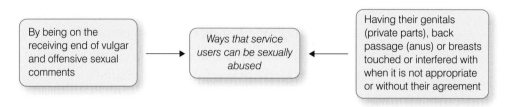

Sexual abuse causes embarrassment, isolation and anxiety. There can also be pain, bleeding and bruising. It denies service users their rights to safety and protection. It shows them no respect, invades their privacy and takes away their dignity.

Emotional abuse

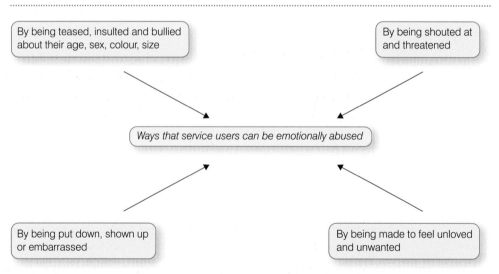

Emotional abuse causes sadness, a feeling of worthlessness and a lack of self-confidence. People who are emotionally abused can find it difficult to show their feelings or affection for anyone else. It denies service users their right to feel emotionally safe and secure. It also demonstrates prejudice and discrimination in the abuser.

Financial abuse

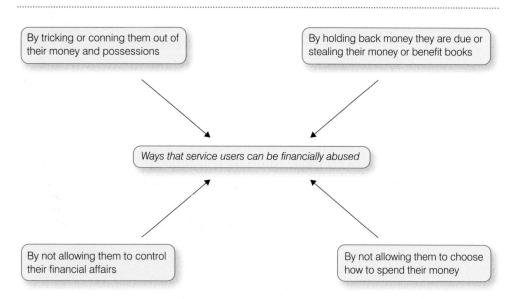

By tricking or conning them out of their money and possessions

By holding back money they are due or stealing their money or benefit books

Ways that service users can be financially abused

By not allowing them to control their financial affairs

By not allowing them to choose how to spend their money

Financial abuse causes a shortage of money and a loss of interest in financial affairs. Service users who are financially abused become worried, depressed and helpless. They are denied respect and the right to privacy and choice. They become dependent and lose the power to run their lives as they want.

Institutional abuse

Institutions are organisations that are set up for a number of reasons, one of which is to provide care services for people in need. Your workplace is an example of an institution. Institutional abuse is where the institution's work procedures and routines become more important than the people being cared for.

Institutional abuse causes service users to lose interest in everything around them. They become sluggish, bored, depressed, lose their self-worth and have feelings of despair and utter hopelessness.

By controlling the way they live, e.g. meals, medication and toileting have to be carried out at certain times

By taking away their independence because it's easier and quicker for staff to do everything for them

Ways that institutions abuse service users

By not allowing them to take part in or make contributions to the running of the organisation where they receive care

By treating them all the same because there isn't time to get to know them as individuals

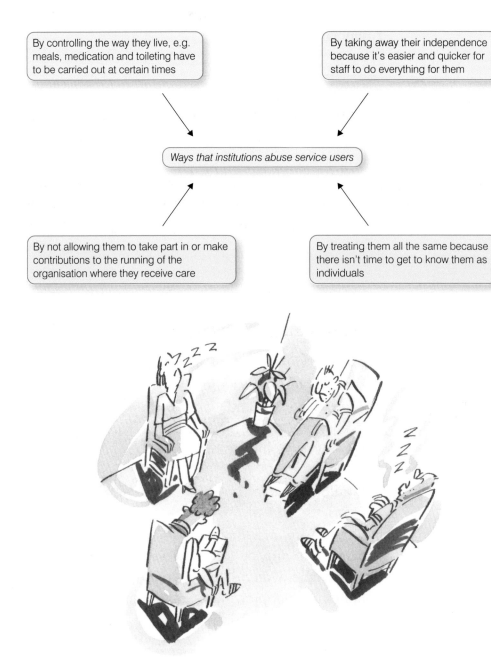

Institutional abuse denies service users their individuality

Treating service users like this – 'institutionalising' them – is not acceptable. It takes away their power, it shows no respect for their individuality, it denies them the right to make choices and to express their views, it doesn't encourage independence and it doesn't foster working partnerships.

CHECK YOUR UNDERSTANDING

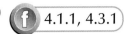 4.1.1, 4.3.1

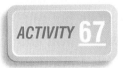

Talk with your colleagues and supervisor about examples of abuse at work, that you have read about in the papers or have seen on the TV. Complete the table to show your understanding of abuse.

Type of abuse: physical, sexual, emotional, financial or institutional?	Signs of abuse: how the individual was affected physically	Symptoms of abuse: how the individual was affected emotionally

9.2 RECOGNISING NEGLECT

Abusive behaviour is usually carried out on purpose to give the abuser a feeling of power. Neglect, on the other hand, is not deliberate but can also have distressing, disturbing and long-lasting effects on physical and emotional health and well-being.

Neglect means failing to care for others. Self-neglect means failing to care for ourselves. We all tend to neglect ourselves from time to time, for example how often have you:

- skipped breakfast because you went to bed late, didn't hear the alarm and were pushed for time?
- spent your last few pounds on treating the children when you needed spoiling more than they did?
- forgotten to make or keep an appointment with the dentist because looking after everybody else seemed more important?.

Neglecting yourself by not getting enough rest, not eating properly and not looking after yourself physically and emotionally will, in due course, have an effect on your health and well-being. Unless you find time to care for yourself, you will become run-down and no longer able to care for others, never mind yourself.

You read in Chapter 3 that some service users neglect themselves and that care workers must remain alert to signs of self-neglect. Service users are already in need of care and self-neglect only makes matters worse for them.

It is your responsibility to remain watchful for signs of self-neglect and to let your supervisor know if you feel that service users are neglecting themselves.

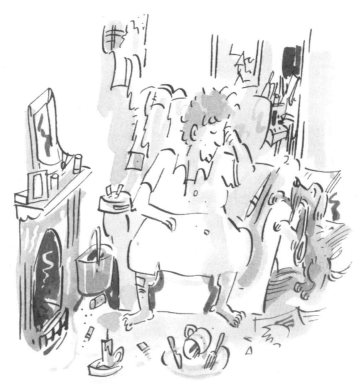

Care workers must look out for signs of self-neglect

How to stay physically and emotionally healthy	The physical signs and emotional symptoms of service users who self-neglect
Eat and drink sensibly	Loss of interest in cooking and eating, weight loss or gain
Maintain good standards of hygiene and appearance	Loss of interest in themselves and how they live: becoming grubby, scruffy and untidy, not dressing appropriately; allowing the living environment to become dirty and smelly
Take prescribed medicines	Physical and mental ill health
Keep warm and comfortable	'Making do' with a cold, damp environment
Stay in contact with family and friends	Becoming lonely and isolated; finding it difficult to mix with others and to make new friends
Stay safe and secure	Health, safety and security risks which can lead to, e.g. physical harm, fire, intruders and theft

Now think about whether you are guilty of neglecting service users:

- do you ever forget to do things you've been asked to do, e.g. take a glass of water to someone who is thirsty, perhaps because you've got too many other things to think about?
- do you ever promise to do something, e.g. help a service user to the toilet, but because you're so busy you don't keep your promise?.

Although you would never neglect service users on purpose, circumstances can mean that it's often all too easy to overlook their requests and needs. But like neglecting yourself, neglecting the care of service users can lead to a down-turn in their physical and mental health and well-being. Thirst can quickly become dehydration and urine-soaked clothing can lead to sores and rashes in addition to a loss of dignity.

You read earlier that abusive behaviour results from not using the values of care in your work with service users. The same can be said about neglect. You will not neglect service users if you show them respect, support their rights and communicate and work with them as individuals. By working with service users in this way, you will also increase their value for themselves and so help reduce the possibility of self-neglect.

CHECK YOUR UNDERSTANDING 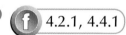 4.2.1, 4.4.1

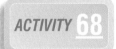

Talk with your colleagues and supervisor about examples of neglect at work, that you have read about in the papers or seen on the TV. Complete the table to show your understanding of neglect.

Type of neglect: self-neglect or neglect by others?	Signs of neglect: how the neglect affected the individual physically	Symptoms of neglect: how the neglect affected the individual emotionally

9.3 RESPONDING TO ABUSE AND NEGLECT

Service users can be abused and neglected by their families, their carers, their care workers, in fact anyone who has contact with them. It is hard to accept that people who are emotionally close to or who work with service users can behave abusively but the reality is they can and they do.

If service users tell you (disclose) that they have been abused or that they are being neglected:

- make sure they understand that you will have to talk to your supervisor about what they tell you – always get help from a senior worker
- make sure they understand that other people might have to be told but only those people who are concerned with their safety
- reassure them that anything they say will be treated with respect and confidentiality
- listen to them and check that you have understood things correctly
- ask 'open' questions that give them an opportunity to give you a full description of what has happened, e.g. 'can you tell me what happened?'
- don't ask 'Yes/No' questions, e.g. 'Did she hit you?' as these won't give you a full story
- show them that you believe them.

If you see someone behaving abusively:

- try to calm things down. Use words, body language and a tone of voice that are soothing and reassuring. Don't make the situation worse by staring at the abuser or using aggressive body language
- ask them very firmly and assertively to stop what they are doing but never threaten or humiliate them or make it difficult for them to back off.

If the abusive behaviour becomes violent and unsafe, your priority is to get yourself and others out of danger and to call for help. Don't try to deal with situations like this until you have more experience.

If you are worried that one of your colleagues is abusing or neglecting service users by not responding to their needs, being rude to them, shouting at them or not respecting their privacy, talk your concerns over with your supervisor. If you are worried that your supervisor is being abusive or neglectful, talk to somebody in a more senior position. Never make accusations unless you have witnessed abuse or neglect or you have evidence to prove your case. Remember, there might be a very good explanation for behaviour that appears to be abusive.

Follow your workplace procedure for recording and reporting neglect and abuse. This means:

- reporting your worries, what you have seen and what you have been told to your supervisor without delay
- recording information in writing as soon as possible, before you forget any details.

Your written accounts of abusive incidents may be needed to be read by your manager, doctors, the police, social workers and so on. So remember that your records must be readable, understandable, relevant, clear, to-the-point, factual and checkable and follow procedures regarding confidentiality.

DEVELOP GOOD WORK PRACTICE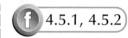

ACTIVITY 69

Read your workplace procedure on neglect and abuse. Make notes on what it tells you about:

- when to report abuse and neglect
- how to report and record abuse and neglect.

_____

_____

_____

_____

_____

_____

_____

_____

_____

_____

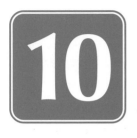

10 Understanding the experiences and particular needs of service users

In Chapter 3 you learned about the needs of service user groups. This chapter aims to develop your understanding of service users as individuals and how their individual life experiences influence their care needs. It also looks at how service users' needs can be met through the delivery of value-based personalised care and why it is sometimes difficult for service providers to deliver care that has been requested.

Successful completion of the activities in this chapter will enable you to demonstrate your understanding of the Foundation Standard *Understand the experiences and particular needs of the individuals using the service*. It will also give you an opportunity to develop evidence for key skills unit Communication at level 1.

What is covered in this chapter?

This chapter contributes to the knowledge and understanding you need for the following NVQ Care unit:
O1 : Foster people's equality, diversity and rights

10.1 UNDERSTANDING THE INDIVIDUAL NEEDS OF SERVICE USERS

Understanding your service users

You might have the same shape of nose and the same eye colour as other members of your family. You might enjoy going to the same places and doing the same things as your friends. However, there is nobody that is absolutely the same as you. Even identical twins are different from each other in many ways.

We are all different because we each have a different genetic make-up from everybody else and because we have each had different life experiences. The sorts of experience that make you an individual include those to do with:

- your family – the only child, the eldest, the youngest and the child from a single-parent family have different experiences of growing up; and you may have experience of being a parent
- your marital status – being married, living with a partner, being divorced and widowed each bring different experiences
- your gender – boys and girls are usually brought up differently and men and women often experience different roles in the family and the workplace
- your education and employment – different people learn different things at school, experience different degrees of success in their studies, and work in jobs with different amounts of pay and importance
- your race and cultural background – people have different experiences according to their skin colour, religion, cultural values and so on

- your social class – people living in run-down areas and poor quality housing and who are on low incomes have very different experiences from people who are higher up the social ladder
- your age – how old you are and the period of time you have lived through affect your views, expectations and knowledge and understanding of life
- your health and ability – people with a long-term illness or a physical disability have very different experiences from people who are healthy and able-bodied.

All these different experiences combine to make us the unique individuals that we are. Because we are all unique, it's no wonder that we all want and expect different things! Service users are equally unique so it follows that they have their own individual wants and expectations. It is your role to be interested in and learn as much as you can about your service users' experiences. When you understand them in this way, you will be better able to care for them appropriately.

> **CASE STUDY: Dennis and Sunil**
>
> *Dennis and Sunil are both in their late seventies and need support with maintaining their appearance, expressing themselves and feeding. Dennis is English and Sunil comes from India. Both have worked all their lives in a London hospital, Dennis as a porter and Sunil as a doctor. Sunil is a widower with three grown up children whereas Dennis has never been married.*

These two gentlemen are alike in that they have similar care needs, they are a similar age and they are both male. However, their very different experiences have made them unique individuals.

Because of their different experiences, Dennis and Sunil are likely to have different expectations of life, including how they wish to be supported. This doesn't mean that they should be given different standards of care. It simply means that the way they are cared for should, as far as is possible, meet their needs in a way that shows respect for their experiences and expectations.

By giving personalised care that takes account of and shows respect for individual experiences and expectations, you will demonstrate that you are using the care values in your work.

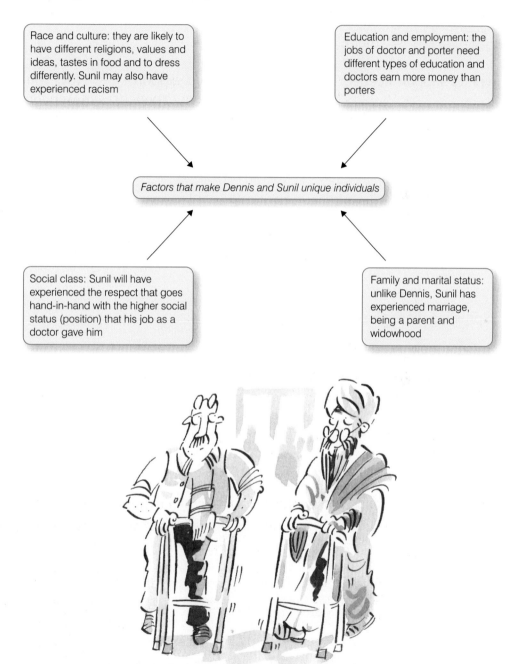

Race and culture: they are likely to have different religions, values and ideas, tastes in food and to dress differently. Sunil may also have experienced racism

Education and employment: the jobs of doctor and porter need different types of education and doctors earn more money than porters

Factors that make Dennis and Sunil unique individuals

Social class: Sunil will have experienced the respect that goes hand-in-hand with the higher social status (position) that his job as a doctor gave him

Family and marital status: unlike Dennis, Sunil has experienced marriage, being a parent and widowhood

Make yourself aware of your service users' different needs

CHECK YOUR UNDERSTANDING 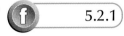 5.2.1

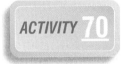 Complete the table to show your understanding of how Dennis and Sunil's different life experiences would affect the way you support them.

Type of support needed	How you would support Dennis	How you would support Sunil
Maintaining appearance		
Expressing themselves		
Feeding		

Understanding your service users' needs

All human beings have the same basic needs.

Basic needs	Examples of basic needs
Physical needs	A nutritious and balanced diet, shelter, a good standard of hygiene, warmth, to be active, protection from disease, safety and security
Intellectual needs	To communicate, to use our minds, to deal with everyday problems
Emotional needs	To be independent, self-confident, to love and to be loved, to be valued and respected and to have a feeling of self-worth
Social needs	To have a sense of belonging, to have relationships and to be able to socialise with friends and family

We all also have specific needs to varying degrees. Service users need support because they have specific needs. Specific needs include:

- physical disabilities resulting from, for instance, a stroke or arthritis
- sensory impairments such as sight or hearing problems
- particular conditions such as dementia and mental health problems.

Having a specific need has a knock-on effect on basic needs. Imagine if you had broken your arm. You would need help with simple everyday activities like eating, drinking, washing and dressing. This would mean losing some independence. Unless you had some help you might have to pull out of social activities, which could result in you feeling bored and lonely. In other words, a broken arm can result in you needing help with a range of physical, intellectual, emotional and social needs.

CASE STUDY: *Mary*

Mary's memory is failing her. She forgets to eat, to dress appropriately for the weather, to take her medication. She forgets what day it is and the names and faces of the people who visit and care for her.

Mary's specific need is to do with her memory loss. However, her memory loss is having a knock-on effect on her basic needs.

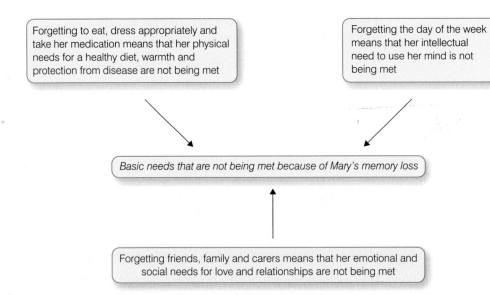

Forgetting to eat, dress appropriately and take her medication means that her physical needs for a healthy diet, warmth and protection from disease are not being met

Forgetting the day of the week means that her intellectual need to use her mind is not being met

Basic needs that are not being met because of Mary's memory loss

Forgetting friends, family and carers means that her emotional and social needs for love and relationships are not being met

Your role is to respond to both basic needs and specific needs created by service users' conditions, impairments or disabilities. And of course, your response must show respect for their individuality and consideration of their expectations of care.

DEVELOP GOOD WORK PRACTICE

 5.2.2

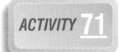

ACTIVITY 71

Talk to your supervisor about the specific care needs (physical disability, sensory impairment or particular condition) of two of your service users. Find out how you should respond to these needs.

Specific care need

How to respond to specific care needs

Service user 1

_____

_____

_____

_____

_____

Service user 2

_____

_____

_____

_____

_____

Responding to the changing needs of service users

Your service users' care needs will have been assessed and written into their care plans. Care plans are exclusive to the service users they are written for and are based on all their physical, intellectual, emotional and social needs. They also take account of their personal expectations about how care should be given.

Care plans spell out how, where and when care will be given. They are agreed by the service user and the organisations that will be delivering the care.

Statutory organisations, e.g. Local Authority Housing, Personal and Social Care Services and National Health Service Trusts. These organisations are required by law to be in existence

Non-statutory independent or private organisations, e.g. private residential and nursing homes, pharmacies, shops that sell aids and adaptations. These organisations are run as businesses to make a profit

Organisations that are involved in the delivery of care

Voluntary, charity and self-help groups e.g. Age Concern, Alzheimer's Society, Royal National Institute for the Blind. These organisations are usually non-profit-making

Informal, unpaid carers, e.g. family, friends, neighbours, church visitors

It is your responsibility to follow care plans exactly as they tell you. Your supervisor will keep a check on how effective you are at following care plans by observing you at work or asking you questions.

You may be asked to tell your supervisor how you have followed a care plan. Alternatively you may have to complete care plans with details of any activities you have carried out. If you do, remember that what you write must be readable, understandable, accurate, checkable and only contain relevant information. It must also be signed and dated.

It is also your responsibility to watch out for changes in service users' needs and circumstances.

Service users' needs	How needs and circumstances can change
Physical needs	They can find it increasingly difficult to move around, to use the toilet or see or hear; their savings can become used up
Intellectual needs	They can become confused and lose interest in the world around them
Emotional needs	They can become withdrawn and depressed
Social needs	They can lose interest in maintaining relationships and contacts and become isolated; also friends and family don't visit as often as they used to

Changes like these are responded to by changes in care plans. The people who are involved in discussing the changes that need to be made (reviewing the care plan) include:

- first and foremost the service user, their family and friends
- the organisations giving the care (including yours)
- others who are interested in and involved with the service user, such as social workers, doctors and nurses.

As a care worker, you have an important role to play in the care plan review process. Because you communicate effectively and work in partnership with your service users, you are in a good position to detect changes in their circumstances and needs and to encourage them to voice their opinions on how their care might be improved.

You may not be involved in care plan review meetings at this stage in your career but it is your responsibility to tell your supervisor if you think service users' circumstances and needs have changed and how you and they think their care can be improved.

DEVELOP GOOD WORK PRACTICE 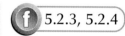 5.2.3, 5.2.4

ACTIVITY 72

Think about one of your service users. Note down:

1 how you know what care to give him or her

_____

_____

_____

2 how you know whether the care you give is effective

_____

_____

_____

3 what you would do if you felt that the care you gave no longer met their needs.

_____

_____

_____

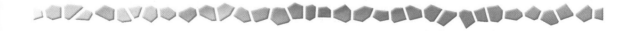

10.2 MEETING THE INDIVIDUAL NEEDS OF SERVICE USERS

The importance of service users in meeting their needs

Good, value-based care practice involves respecting service users' views about what their care needs are and how they wish to be cared for. In other words, it means putting service users at the heart or centre of the process of planning and delivering their care. Services that see service users as being central to their care are called 'user-led' care.

CASE STUDY: Rabeena

Rabeena is a resident in a home for elderly people. She doesn't see as well as she used to and as a result is losing her confidence and becoming withdrawn.

How could you support Rabeena? Because she should be central to decisions about her care, you would first of all discuss with her the type of care she wants and how she wants it to be given. What sort of care do you think she and you might discuss?

- a visit to an optician to see whether there is any medical problem with her eyes or whether new glasses would help?
- a magnifying glass, 'talking' books and large print newspapers and magazines?
- asking charities set up to help people with sight impairments for information about aids such as a white stick?
- getting together with others who have a similar problem to find out how they cope?

Listen to service users' requests for care and keep your supervisor informed about their wishes. As a result of your discussion with Rabeena, the services of an optician, a care aids retailer, the local library, a charity and a self-help group could be requested. These organisations would meet Rabeena's specific need for help due to her failing sight.

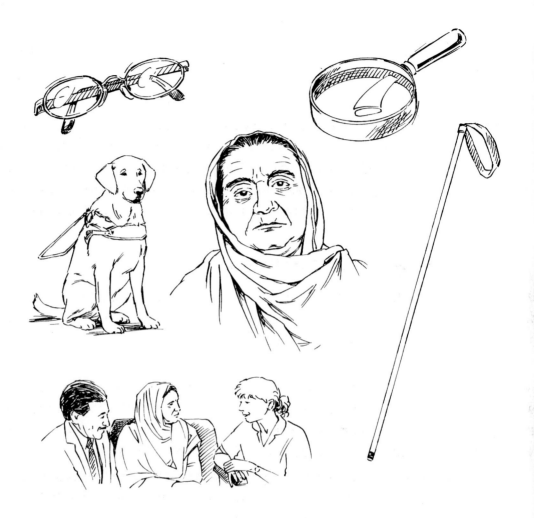

They would also meet some of Rabeena's basic needs:

- the optician will check the health of her eyes and a white stick could help her to move around with safety (physical needs)
- a magnifying glass, large print and 'talking' books will help her to read and listen and keep her mind active (intellectual need)
- talking with other people would give her an opportunity to mix and to boost her confidence (social and emotional needs).

Care that meets all a service user's individual needs is known as <u>holistic care</u>. Caring for service users holistically means you are using the values of care in your work. In particular it enables you to show that you recognise them as unique individuals with their own basic and specific needs.

191

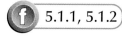

What do you think?

ACTIVITY 73

Think of one of your service users. Jot down how you ensure that:

- s/he is central to the care that you give
- you care for him/her in a holistic way.

_____

_____

_____

_____

_____

_____

_____

_____

_____

_____

Problems in meeting service users' needs

It isn't always easy to satisfy service users' requests for care. For example:

- care is requested at a certain hospital or day centre but transport or disabled facilities aren't available
- care is requested as soon as possible but there is a waiting list.

It could also be the case that requests for care aren't practical for care service providers. For example:

- it might not be possible for visits or appointments to be made at the time preferred by the service user or for a chosen doctor to make a visit
- it might be felt that the care requested is too expensive or wouldn't be effective.

Care service providers – including your employer – are constrained by having a limited number of staff, restricted resources (e.g. equipment, beds, funds) and only 24 hours in the day. How many times have you wished you had another pair of legs or more time!

If there is a conflict between service users' preferences and the care that can be provided for them, talk with them and the care team about possible alternatives. The aim is for an agreement to be reached about what is best for everyone.

DEVELOP GOOD WORK PRACTICE 5.1.3

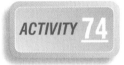 **ACTIVITY 74**

Talk with your supervisor about how to deal with problems you might experience in meeting service users' requests for care. Complete the table to show your understanding.

Problems in meeting service users' needs	How these problems can be dealt with

The importance of non-judgmental care

You read earlier about how different life experiences combine to make us individual in the ways we think and behave. For example, you might have been brought up to shrug off minor illnesses such as coughs and colds. Because of this you never let poor health stop you doing what you want. But a colleague might have been brought up to take herself off to bed every time she felt under the weather. Now she and her children take time off work and school whenever they are off colour.

How do you judge people who think and behave differently from you? Your friends probably think and behave much the same as you and you chose each other as friends for this reason! Having things in common makes for good relationships. What about your service users? It's unlikely that they will have much so much in common with you. Does this mean that you judge them in a negative way, i.e. that you are prejudiced against them?

It can be difficult for care workers not to make negative judgements about service users. You might have different views about skin colour, sexual behaviour and sexual preferences, mental health, social class, child rearing and responsibility for elderly relatives. You may have different values, standards of personal hygiene, appearance and table manners and there may be differences in the way you use language. Whatever the differences are, it is not your role to make judgements.

Making negative judgements about service users means that you will find it difficult to communicate and develop effective working relationships with them. You may start to discriminate against them and treat them less fairly than other service users. Being discriminated against can make people feel unimportant, worthless, frustrated and angry. As you now know, discrimination flies in the face of good, value-led care practice.

If you are worried that differences in views and behaviour are affecting your care work, talk things over with your supervisor. Be open to suggestions as to how you might change your beliefs and expectations of people's behaviour. You're never too old to learn!

What do you think?

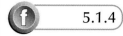

5.1.4

ACTIVITY 75

Think about a service user whose views and behaviours make it difficult for you to work with them. Note down:

1 how you treat them as a result of the way you feel about them

_____

_____

_____

_____

_____

_____

2 how your treatment of them might affect them.

_____

_____

_____

_____

_____

_____

Suggested reading

TEXTBOOKS

Clarke, L., *Health and Social Care for Foundation GNVQ*, Stanley Thornes, 2000

Clarke, L., Rowell, K. and White, M., *An Entry Level Course in Caring*, Nelson Thornes, 2002

Clarke, L., Rowell, K. and White, M., *First Course on Caring*, Nelson Thornes, 1993

Trickett, J., *The Prevention of Food Poisoning*, Nelson Thornes, 2001

Wells, J. *The Home Care Worker's Handbook*, UKHCA, 1999

LEAFLETS

Areas of Risk – Home Hygiene, Domestos

Avoiding Slips, Trips and Broken Hips, Department of Trade and Industry, 1999

COSHH: The New Brief Guide for Employers, Health and Safety Executive, INDG136L

Electrical Safety Leads to Fire Safety, Home Office, FL04

Employee's Guide to the Health and Safety at Work Act, Scriptographic Publications

Everyone's Guide to RIDDOR 95, Health and Safety Executive, 1995

Falls – How to Avoid Them and How to Cope, Age Concern/Royal Society for the Prevention of Accidents

Fire Kills – You Can Prevent It. Get a Plan Get Out Alive, Home Office

First Aid – Basic Advice on First Aid at Work, Health and Safety Executive

Food Safety and Temperature Control, Foodlink

Get the Balance Right, British Meat Nutrition Education Service

Getting to Grips with Manual Handling, Health and Safety Executive

A Guide to the General Food Hygiene Regulations 1995 – Food Safety, Department of Health

How to Choose and Use Fire Extinguishers for the Home, Home Office

In Doubt? Keep Them Out, Home Office

Preventing Slips, Trips and Falls at Work, Health and Safety Executive

Safe as Houses, Department of Health

A Safer Place Self-audit Tool – Combating Violence Against Social Care Staff, Department of Health, 2001

Safety and Security at Home Age Concern England

A Short Guide to the Personal Protective Equipment at Work Regs 1992, Health and Safety Executive

So You Think You're Safe at Home? Department of Trade and Industry/Royal Society for the Prevention of Accidents

Stay Safe at Home, Department of Trade and Industry

Step Up to Safety, Department of Trade and Industry

The Health Guide, Health Promotion England

Violence at Work, Health and Safety Executive

Working Alone in Safety, Health and Safety Executive

SPECIALIST MAGAZINES AND JOURNALS

Nursing and Residential Care

Primary Healthcare

Care and Health

Working with Older People

Homecare Professional

Health and Social Care in the Community

Caring Today

Community Care

Community Nurse

Disability and Society

Health and Hygiene

USEFUL WEBSITES

www.topss.org.uk – Training Organisation for the Personal Social Services

www.socialcareassoc.com – The Social Care Association

www.skillsforhealth.org.uk – Training Organisation for the Health Care Sector

www.nhs.uk – The National Health Service

www.hmso.gov.uk/acts/acts2000 – Care Standards Act

www.doh.gov.uk/ncsc – Department of Health Care Homes for Older People: National Minimum Standards

www.carestandards.org.uk – The National Care Standards Commission

www.doh.gov.uk/COS – Department of Health – Children, Older People and Social Care

www.ncha.gb.com – National Care Homes Association

www.learndirect-futures.co.uk/job_profiles – Job profiles, including those in care

www.doh.gov.uk/violencetaskforce/audit.htm – Department of Health – A Safer Place Self-audit Tool – Combating Violence Against Social Care Staff, Department of Health

www.ace.org.uk – Age Concern England

www.pcaw.co.uk – Public Concern at Work, Whistleblowing

Glossary

Advocacy
Speaking for or acting on behalf of a service user.

Alzheimer's disease
A form of brain disease that causes gradually increasing confusion, loss of memory and inability to think properly.

Arthritis
Inflamed, swollen joints.

Asphyxiation
Inability to breath, suffocation.

Cardiac arrest
When the heart stops beating.

Carers
People who care for a family member, friend or neighbour on a voluntary, unpaid basis. They are sometimes called 'informal carers'.

Care plan
A plan to provide care services to an individual (or family). The plan follows an assessment or review of the individual's (or family's) needs and involves service users, their family and carers and relevant professionals.

Care package
A group of services brought together to achieve the care plan.

Care service provider
The organisation responsible for providing care services e.g. the owners and managers of a residential home.

Care setting
The place where care is provided and in which a care worker works. This could be a residential care home, a day care centre or the service user's own home.

Care team
The people who have a responsibility for the care of an individual including the person himself.

Care values
Care values are the values or beliefs that underpin or shape care work. Use of the care values by a care worker demonstrates good work practice.

Care workers	People who are employed to care for service users. They are sometimes called 'formal carers'.
Challenging behaviour	Behaviour which can range from demanding and difficult through to offensive, threatening and violent.
Confidentiality	Confidentiality is about respecting service users right to privacy and being careful about what information is passed on and who it is passed on to.
Contagious disease	A disease that is passed from one person to another by body contact.
Dementia	A condition where a service user is confused and has a problem with, for example, short-term memory or communication.
Discrimination	Treating people unfairly because of the way they look or behave.
Hazardous	Dangerous.
Holistic care	Caring for someone in an holistic way means meeting all their care needs – physical, emotional, intellectual and social.
Impetigo	A skin infection caused by bacteria and usually found on the faces of children.
Infection	A disease that can be caught from an infected person or object.
Intervertebral disc	One of the round, flat pads of tissue that separates each bone of the backbone from the next one and allows the backbone to bend.
Labelling	Describing people by characteristics such as their appearance or behaviour.
Ligament	A strip or sheet of stretchy tissue that connects the bones of the skeleton together.
Mobility problems	The condition of having difficulty moving around because of restricted use of the legs and feet.
NVQ	National Vocational Qualification.

Oppression	Harsh, cruel, controlling treatment.
Pelvis	The ring of bones at the bottom of body to which the legs are attached.
Pneumonia	Infection of the lungs.
Prejudice	Judging people without knowing or understanding them.
Pressure sores	The condition that results from pressure or friction on the skin.
Ringworm	A fungal infection of the skin, often of the scalp, where it causes the hair to fall out in patches. It is very infectious and can be caught from animals such as cows and sheep.
Risk assessment	A check to see whether an activity could cause an injury and how the risk of injury could be reduced.
Service users	The people the service is helping. This includes the people being cared for and their family and friends.
Service user groups	These are groups of people who have similar care needs, such as older people, children and people with mental health problems.
Spinal cord	The bundle of nerves, running inside the backbone, that connects the brain with the rest of the body and controls movement and feeling in the whole of the body below the neck.
Statutory Organisations	Organisations that the law requires to be in place e.g. National Health Service Trusts, Local Authority Social Services Departments.
Stereotyping	A way of thinking about people because of the way they look or behave.
Tetanus	A serious infection of the brain caused by bacteria that normally live in the soil. It causes

	the muscles to go into spasm and 'seize up'.
Thrush	An infection, usually occurring in babies' mouths but sometimes in the vagina in adult women, with white, creamy patches of a fungus called *Candida albicans*.
TOPSS	The National Training Organisation for the Personal and Social Services.
TOPSS England	The branch of TOPSS that sets standards for training in England.
Tuberculosis	An infection, usually of the lungs, that causes high temperature, sweating, serious weight loss and often death.
User-led care	User-led care is where service users are involved in the assessment of their care needs and in the delivery and review of their care.
Vertebra	One of the bones of the spine (plural **vertebrae**).

Index